An Atlas of
PSORIASIS

THE ENCYCLOPEDIA OF VISUAL MEDICINE SERIES

An Atlas of
PSORIASIS

Lionel Fry

St. Mary's Hospital
London

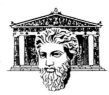

The Parthenon Publishing Group
International Publishers in Medicine, Science & Technology

Casterton Hall, Carnforth,
Lancs, LA6 2LA, UK

120 Mill Road, Park Ridge,
New Jersey 07656, USA

British Library Cataloguing-in-Publication Data
Fry, L.
    Atlas of Psoriasis. – (Encyclopedia of Visual Medicine
Series)
    I. Title   II. Series
    616.5
    ISBN 1-85070-410-4

Library of Congress Cataloging-in-Publication Data
Fry, Lionel.
    An atlas of psoriasis/ L. Fry.
        p.   cm. – – (The Encyclopedia of visual medicine series)
    Includes bibliographical references and index.
    ISBN 1-85070-410-4
    1. Psoriasis – – Atlases.   I. Title.   II. Series.
    [DNLM: 1. Psoriasis – – atlases.   WR 17 F946a]
RL 321.F79   1992
616.5'26 – – dc20
DNLM/DLC
for Library of Congress   92-11856
                                                         CIP

Published in the UK and Europe by
The Parthenon Publishing Group Limited
Casterton Hall, Carnforth
Lancs. LA6 2LA

Published in North America by
The Parthenon Publishing Group Inc.
120 Mill Road
Park Ridge
New Jersey 07656, USA

Copyright © 1992 Parthenon Publishing Group Ltd

First published 1992

Typeset by AMA Graphics Ltd., Preston
Printed and bound in Spain

Contents

The Encyclopedia of Visual Medicine Series

Titles currently planned in this series include:

An Atlas of Oncology

An Atlas of Hypertension

An Atlas of Common Diseases

An Atlas of Osteoporosis

An Atlas of the Menopause

An Atlas of Contraception

An Atlas of Endometriosis

An Atlas of Ultrasonography in Obstetrics and Gynecology

An Atlas of Practical Radiology

An Atlas of Sexually Transmitted Diseases

An Atlas of Psoriasis

An Atlas of Trauma Management

Series Foreword

The art of effective diagnosis is one that relies to a considerable degree – although certainly not exclusively – on the recognition of visual signs and manifestations of disease. The objective of the Series is to provide a practical aid to diagnosis by illustrating and explaining the wide range of visual signs that a physician needs to be aware of in current medical practice.

Whilst the visual manifestations of disease themselves remain constant, the development of new techniques of invasive and non-invasive diagnosis mean that new images are frequently being added to the range of visual material that the diagnostician must be familiar with: ultrasound, radiology, magnetic resonance imaging, endoscopy and photomicrography all provide examples of this kind of material. It is the intention of this Series to document, where appropriate, the result of such techniques and to explain and elucidate their relevance – in addition to documenting all the more standard visual images.

The Series is also distinctive in that individual volumes will focus on carefully selected, specific topics, which can be covered in some detail – rather than on generalized and broadly-based subject areas that could not easily be covered so thoroughly.

The authors contributing to the Series have all been selected for their special expertise in their own chosen fields, their access to outstanding visual material and their ability to explain the significance of it in an effective and lucid way. Finally, particular emphasis is being placed on achieving a very high quality of colour reproduction in the printing process itself in order to do full justice to the wide variety of visual images presented.

It is hoped that this carefully structured and systematic approach to the visually significant aspects of medicine will make a valuable and ongoing contribution to good diagnostic practice.

Introduction

Psoriasis is a common skin disorder with a world-wide distribution but is commoner in the Caucasians of the western world. So far, the disease has retained its secrets of what actually causes the psoriatic lesion; whilst considerable advances have been made in its management in recent years, there is no absolute cure, and no simple, safe and invariably effective treatment. The first description of psoriasis is credited to Celsus (25 BC–AD 45), but Hippocrates (460–375 BC) probably did see psoriasis, under his heading of 'scaly eruptions', and called them lopoi (from *lepo*, to scale). Galen (AD 133–200) was the first to use the word 'psoriasis' (taken from the Greek word *psora* – the itch). However, from the description of the rash given by Galen, he was probably describing seborrhoeic eczema (scaling and itching of the eyelids). Celsus, in his description of the disease as it is recognized today, described the disease under the term 'impetigo' (from *impeto*, to attack). Thus, from the outset, it would appear that the wrong names were given to skin disorders which are recognized today. Until the end of the eighteenth century, psoriasis and leprosy were grouped together, and psoriatics often faced the same fate as lepers in the fourteenth century, being burnt at the stake. The clinical patterns of psoriasis, as we know them today, were first described by Willan at the beginning of the nineteenth century and the disorder was separated from leprosy in 1841 by the Austrian dermatologist, Hebra.

Section I   A Review of Psoriasis

Epidemiology and histology

The incidence of psoriasis has been estimated by census studies and postal questionnaires, and the reliability of some of the studies is open to question. The highest reported incidences have been in Denmark (2.9%) and the Faroe Isles (2.8%). The average for northern Europe (including the UK) has been given as 2.0%, and Northern Europe is generally considered as having the highest incidence. The incidence in the USA is 1.4%. There appears to be a higher incidence in East, as opposed to West, Africans, and this may explain the low incidence in the Negroes in America. The Arabs have been reported to have an incidence similar to that of the Northern Europeans. There is a low incidence in the Asians of China and the Far East, the incidence in China being reported as 0.37%. The results for the Indian subcontinent have been variable: some studies give a lower incidence than in Europeans, whilst others have reported a similar incidence. The disease is said to be non-existent in the American Indians, and the Aborigines from Samoa. However, the reliability of most of these studies is questionable, apart from those carried out in Northern Europe. The general impression is that the highest incidence is in Europeans, and the lowest in Asians from the East.

The two characteristic features of psoriasis are epidermal hyperplasia and an inflammatory cell infiltrate in both the dermis and epidermis.

In the initial stages, there is slight epidermal hyperplasia with thickening of the rete ridges. The epidermal cells increase in size and there is enlargement of the nucleus, dilatation of the intercellular spaces and infiltration with lymphocytes and macrophages. At a later stage, there is infiltration with polymorphonuclear leukocytes. As the lesion progresses, the epidermal cells show lack of differentiation and further increase in size and number. The granular layer begins to disappear and abnormal parakeratosis appears. This is loosely-bound keratin within which is found degenerative neutrophils. Exudation of neutrophils into the epidermis leads to accumulation of these cells in the upper epidermis, where small micro-abscesses form. In the dermis, there is enlargement and tortuosity of the capillaries, which migrate upwards into the dermal papillae. There is an infiltrate of lymphocytes, particularly around dermal capillaries in the deep papillary network, and, to a lesser extent, of macrophages and occasional neutrophils.

In established psoriasis (Figures 1–3), there is elongation and thickening of the rete ridges, elongation and oedema of the dermal papillae, absent, or a poorly formed, granular layer, parakeratosis, microabscess in the epidermis, enlargement of the capillaries, and a mainly lymphocytic infiltrate around the subpapillary vessels. The basal layer shows an increase of mitotic figures. The re-arrangement of the basement membrane configuration results in its considerable lengthening, due to the elongation of the rete ridges. This feature is characteristic of hyperplasia of the epidermal cells. In fact, other features, such as elongation and dilatation of the capillary loops, and swelling and elongation of the dermal papillae, are also adjustments that have to be made in the architecture of the skin to sustain the increase in cell numbers and their increased metabolic activity. The absent granular layer and abnormal keratin layer (parakeratosis) are probably due to a maturation defect of the rapidly proliferating keratinocytes. Thus, it is possible that the fault in psoriasis is one of rapidly dividing epidermal cells and the histological features are secondary to this proliferation. What stimulates the epidermal cells to proliferate is discussed in the section on aetiology.

In pustular psoriasis, the neutrophils accumulate in greater numbers within the epidermis to form a macro-abscess. What initiates this rare process is unknown, but it is probably related to an increase in neutrophil chemotactic factors.

Prognosis

It is difficult to give a true incidence of the remission rate of psoriasis, as a large population of individuals with slight clinical involvement do not attend dermatological clinics, or even any doctor. Thus, most studies of the natural history are based on results from specialist centres where the more severe forms of the disease are seen. Psoriasis tends to run a variable course; it may have spontaneous remissions which are temporary or permanent, therapy-induced remissions, which again may be temporary or permanent, or it may run a persistent course. The interval of time between the episodes of psoriasis, in those who have remissions, may vary from a few months to several years.

In reported studies, the figures for permanent remission are not favourable. In one study of patients followed up for 21 years (but in which only 84% were available for continuous assessment), 71% had persistent lesions, 13% were free of the disease, and 16% had intermittent lesions. In a study of 30 000 inhabitants of the Faroe Isles over a 20-year period, similar results were obtained: at follow-up after 5 years 17%, after 10 years 14%, and after 20 years 6% were disease-free. However, 48% of the patients had a remission during the 20-year follow-up. Another study, of 5000 patients in the USA, reported that 39% of the patients had a remission which varied from 1 to 84 years. It is difficult to give a firm prognosis to patients with psoriasis because of the variable course. However, a number of clinical features tend to imply a poor outlook; these include early onset, that is under the age of 10 years, extensive and persistent disease, and disease which begins on the face and trunk. Psoriasis which begins after the age of 25 tends to have a better prognosis. Erythrodermic and generalized pustular psoriasis have a poor prognosis, with the disease tending to be severe and persistent. Localized pustular psoriasis is a persistent disorder with over two-thirds of patients having the disease for more than 10 years. Guttate psoriasis usually has a good prognosis, particularly in children. The disease tends to resolve after 3 months. However, in one study of 44 patients, 68% had reportedly developed chronic plaque psoriasis within 1 year of their first attack of guttate psoriasis, and thus the prognosis may not be as good as originally thought.

The prognosis is related to what may be described as 'disease activity'. There appear to be central factors controlling psoriasis as well as local ones. The more active the disease, the poorer the prognosis. Active disease is difficult to clear and relapses quickly after cessation of treatment. The biological factors controlling 'disease activity' are not yet known. However, clinically active disease is associated with appearance of new lesions and extensive involvement. Disease which is inactive undergoes spontaneous resolution. Disease activity may change in time within an individual patient and this adds to the uncertainty in trying to give a firm prognosis.

Genetics

Family studies

It has been known for many years that psoriasis has a hereditary basis, as it was noted that the disease tended to run in families. The early observations supporting an inherited factor were derived from family studies. One of the earliest was in a closed community in a small town in Germany, conducted over a 30-year period. It was found at the beginning of the study that 34% of patients with psoriasis had a positive family history; 5 years later this number had increased to 39%, and at the end of the 30 years it was 56%. Some studies of families with psoriasis through three and four generations strongly support the concept of Mendelian dominance with incomplete penetration, as every affected child had an affected parent. However, other family studies through a similar number of generations did not find that all affected individuals with psoriasis had an affected parent, and asymptomatic carriers were assumed. These latter studies considered that the inheritance was autosomal dominant with 60% penetration. The most recent studies have considered inheritance to be multifactorial, implying that the cause of the disease is due to the effect of several genes, each with a small effect, with a permissive role being played by one, or possibly a few, major genes.

Census studies

There have been two classical census studies: one in the Faroe Isles which studied 30 000 individuals, and another in Sweden which covered 40 000. In the latter, it was found that 6.4% of relatives of patients with psoriasis were affected, compared to 1.96% of the general population. In the study in the closed community in the Faroe Isles, 91% of patients with psoriasis had a family history. This high figure was probably due to the special circumstances of the closed community. Analysis of the data in these two census studies supports the current concept that in psoriasis there is multifactorial inheritance and that simple monogeneic types of inheritance are now excluded.

Twin studies

These strongly support the role of inheritance in psoriasis, as the concordance in monozygotic twins is 65–70%, whilst that for dizygotic twins is 15–20%. Twin studies have also shown that the clinical type of psoriasis, age of onset, the course and severity are determined to a large extent by genetic factors.

Human leukocyte antigens

Early studies of the Class I human leukocyte antigens (HLA) have shown an association with B13, B17 and B37, and genetic linkage has been shown to exist between these antigens. However, the association of these antigens, although significant, is considerably weaker than in some other diseases which have HLA associations, such as ankylosing spondylitis, dermatitis herpetiformis, and insulin-dependent diabetes. Subsequent studies have shown an association with the Class I antigen CW6 and Class II antigen DR7. It is now thought that the primary association for the Class I antigen is with CW6, and that the association with B13, B17 and B37 is due to linkage disequilibrium between these antigens. Thus, there appear to be two susceptibility psoriasis genes, one in the C region (CW6-associated), and the other in the DR region (DR7-associated). However, not all patients have these markers and thus there is genetic variation between populations with psoriasis.

HLA associations and clinical features have also been reported. Early onset of the disease is associated with CW6, which is in linkage disequilibrium with B13, B17 and B37, whilst late onset is associated with CW2 and B27. B13 and B17 are higher in patients with guttate compared to chronic plaque psoriasis, and B13 patients have a higher risk of post-streptococcal flares of their plaque psoriasis. Patients with flexural psoriasis do not have an association with CW6, B13 and B17. This is further support for the suggestion that the clinical patterns of psoriasis are genetically predetermined.

There has been long been an argument as to whether localized palmar/plantar pustular psoriasis is part of the general psoriatic spectrum, or whether it is a separate clinical entity. B13, B17 and B37 have not been found to be raised in localized palmar/plantar pustular psoriasis, thus implying that, genetically, it is distinct from psoriasis. In addition, AW19 and BW35 have been reported to be raised in localized pustular psoriasis but not in plaque psoriasis.

The only other sites of involvement in psoriasis are the joints. However, only a small proportion of patients with skin lesions develop an arthropathy, but the arthropathy may occur without skin lesions. Thus, different predisposing factors may be operative in the expression of the skin and joint lesions. In patients with psoriatic arthropathy, an increase in A26, B38 and DR4 has been found, and, in those patients with sacro-iliitis, there is an increase of B27. Patients who develop erosive arthritis have an increase of DR3. Thus, different HLA associations are found in patients who have the joint compared to the skin lesions, supporting the concept that different genetic factors are important in determining the clinical features. In summary, psoriasis appears to be a genetically determined disorder, with a multifactorial inheritance. However, environmental trigger factors are also likely to play a role in the expression of the disease, and this may explain why the disease may miss generations. Because of this mode of inheritance, and the variable environmental factors, it is difficult to predict the risk of psoriasis in genetic counselling. However, the following is an estimated percentage risk (ter Haar, B. (1986). In Mier, P. D. and van de Kerkof, P. C. M. (eds.) *Textbook of Psoriasis*, p. 11. (Churchill Livingstone)): both parents, 50%; one parent 10%; one sibling 7%; one parent and one sibling 16%; second-degree relative 4%; third-degree relative 1–2%.

Aetiology

Environmental triggers

Although there is undoubtedly a genetic component to the development of psoriasis, environmental factors are also important, and may trigger the disease.

Physical trauma

In approximately one-third of patients with psoriasis, trauma to the skin will result in the development of psoriatic lesions at the site of trauma. This phenomenon was first noted by a physician named Koebner in 1872, and it is now known as the Koebner phenomenon. The nature of the injury is immaterial (Koebner himself described the simultaneous development of psoriasis, in an individual, at the sites of a horsefly bite, a tattoo, bacterial infection and excoriations from horse riding). Although one-third of patients with psoriasis develop lesions after injury to the skin (Koebner-positive), two-thirds do not (Koebner-negative). The Koebner phenomenon is 'all or nothing', that is patients who are Koebner-positive at one site, are positive everywhere, and those who are negative are negative at all sites. This implies that there is a central factor which influences the development of psoriasis. However, patients may transfer from a state of Koebner positivity to negativity, and vice versa; thus, the central factor influencing the development of psoriasis is variable. It has been shown that the injury inducing psoriasis in a Koebner-positive patient must cause epidermal damage. This injury is likely to produce a cytokine cascade, which triggers psoriasis (see section on pathogenesis). The inhibitory factor which stops the development of psoriasis is likely to be part of an immune response and is possibly related to CD8 (suppressor) T lymphocytes.

A recently described phenomenon is the 'reverse Koebner'. In this situation, removal of part of a psoriatic plaque, by shaving through the plaque in the upper dermis, results in that area being replaced by normal-looking skin unaffected by psoriasis. The reverse Koebner and true Koebner are mutually exclusive, that is patients who are Koebner-positive are positive at all sites and cannot exhibit the reverse Koebner, whilst those who show the reverse Koebner do so at all sites and the Koebner phenomenon cannot be induced.

Infections

The organism most commonly associated with psoriasis is the β-haemolytic streptococcus. The original observations were made some 50 years ago when it was noted that tonsillitis often preceded the first appearance of psoriasis. It was subsequently shown that, in patients with psoriasis, there was a significantly higher incidence of a positive streptococcal agglutination test, compared to patients with other skin diseases. The clinical association of guttate psoriasis and streptococcal infections is much stronger than similar infections and plaque psoriasis. Either one or more of the following are present in over half of the patients with guttate psoriasis: history of a sore throat; a positive throat swab for β-haemolytic streptococcus; and a raised antistreptolysin titre. Confirmation of a streptococcal infection in all patients with guttate psoriasis may be difficult because the patients are usually seen a few weeks after the infection, and the antistreptolysin test is not always positive after infection. Further evidence of the role of the streptococcal infections in patients with guttate psoriasis is that circulating T lymphocytes display increased reactivity to streptococcal antigens, compared to control subjects. This implies that there may be T lymphocytes which respond selectively to streptococcal antigens. T cells are now thought to play a central role in the pathogenesis of psoriasis (see below), and it is possible that streptococcal antigens are the trigger in the skin which initiates the psoriatic process.

The role of streptococcal infections in the more common form of psoriasis, chronic plaque, is less certain. However, some studies have shown that the majority of patients with guttate psoriasis do eventually progress to chronic plaque disease, so it might be argued that, in this instance, the streptococcus did initiate the disease. Recent studies on peripheral blood lymphocytes have also shown a high incidence of circulating T cells reactive with streptococcal antigens, implying there are T cells which respond specifically to the streptococcus. As in guttate psoriasis, they may be responsible for initiating and maintaining the psoriatic process in the skin.

Apart from the streptococcus, there is often a history of other infections prior to the outbreak or deterioration of psoriasis. These include viral and other bacterial infections, but the evidence for another specific organism initiating psoriasis is lacking at the present time. Human immunodeficiency virus (HIV) infection has been reported to exacerbate psoriasis. It is known that the virus invades Langerhans cells and these cells then become activated, possibly enhancing the psoriatic process. A possible direct stimulatory effect on keratinocytes has also been suggested.

Stress

There is no doubt that, in patients with the genetic predisposition for psoriasis, stress may precipitate psoriasis and aggravate existing disease. However, the widely held view by patients that psoriasis is due to 'nerves' is not correct. The proportion of patients with psoriasis, in whom stress plays an important role as a trigger, is difficult to estimate because of the problems of defining stress and because various stressful situations affect individuals differently, depending on their personality. Studies on the grade of neuroticism in patients with psoriasis have not shown any difference compared to a control group.

How stress induces or aggravates psoriasis is not known. Stress has effects on hormones, the autonomic nervous and immune systems. There is now accumulating evidence that the immune system is involved in disease expression and this may lead to alteration in the homeostatic mechanisms which control epidermal proliferation, the hallmark of psoriasis.

Drugs

Certain drugs, notably lithium, β-blockers, antimalarials (chloroquin, hydroxychloroquin and quinacrine), and non-steroidal anti-inflammatory drugs, have been reported to aggravate psoriasis. How these different drugs with different chemical structures can have the same effect is difficult to explain; they may affect the psoriatic process at different stages but with the same results. Steroids, both systemic and topical, have a beneficial effect on psoriasis, but withdrawal of systemic steroids (and occasionally potent topical steroids) may result in flare-up of psoriasis, and, for this reason, systemic steroids tend not to be used in the treatment of psoriasis.

Hypocalcaemia

It is an interesting observation that the very rare condition of hypocalcaemia aggravates psoriasis. This observation may be of importance in unravelling the pathogenetic pathway of the psoriatic process, particularly as vitamin D, both orally and topically, improves psoriasis.

Alcohol

There has long been a reported association between psoriasis and a high intake of alcohol. Originally this was attributed to patients taking alcohol in an attempt to alleviate their feelings of frustration and anxiety/depression because of their psoriasis. However, more recent studies have shown a deleterious effect of alcohol on the psoriatic process, but the mechanism has to be elucidated.

Climate

Psoriasis tends to improve in warm climates and to become worse in cold ones. This seems to be independent of the effects of ultraviolet light. This effect of climate on psoriasis may partly explain the high incidence of the disease in the northern European countries.

Pathogenesis

Immunopathology

It was known well over 100 years ago that the two main histological factors of psoriasis were epidermal hyperplasia and an inflammatory cell infiltrate in the dermis. It was also suggested that infection may precipitate the disease. Even at that time there was argument as to whether the epidermal hyperplasia or the inflammatory cell infiltrate was the primary event in psoriasis. In this century, up until the 1980s, the primary fault in psoriasis was considered to be epidermal hyperplasia. It was argued that genetic abnormality led to an inherent defect of the cell cycle of the keratinocyte, which led to epidermal proliferation. Other suggestions as to the cause of psoriasis have been of a specific biochemical defect, including abnormality of cyclic AMP, arachidonic acid and its metabolites, polyamines, proteases and antiproteases, and in a variety of intracellular enzymes. However, all the abnormalities described could just as well be secondary to psoriasis rather than the cause, and to date none of these abnormalities has been shown to be the primary defect in psoriasis.

Recent studies over the last decade have now shown that psoriasis is probably mediated by immunological mechanisms, and that the inflammatory cell infiltrate is probably the primary event and the hyperplasia secondary. These observations have been possible because of the advent of monoclonal antibodies, which have allowed the mapping of immunological pathways.

Initial studies on peripheral blood lymphocytes showed that, in patients with extensive psoriasis, there was a decrease in both total and CD4 (helper) T cells. Studies on the skin showed that the inflammatory cell infiltrate was mainly T lymphocytes of the CD4 subset (T helper cells), although some were of the CD8 subset (T suppressor cells). In addition, the CD4/CD8 ratio was greater in the skin than the blood. Taken together, these observations imply a selective recruitment of CD4 cells into the skin in psoriasis.

Unfortunately, there is no animal model for psoriasis, but guttate psoriasis is an acute, self-limiting form of the disease and allows the evolution to be studied. Using guttate psoriasis as a model, it has been shown that, in the early stages, there is an influx of T lymphocytes, both CD4 and CD8, into the epidermis, but only the CD4 cells are activated. These activated CD4 cells are found in close apposition to the dendritic processes of the antigen-presenting cells (the Langerhans cells) (Figure 4). During resolution of psoriasis, there is a further influx of T cells into the epidermis, but at this stage no activated CD4 cells are found, all the activated T cells being CD8. These activated CD8 T cells are also found in close apposition to the dendritic processes of the Langerhans cells (Figure 5). As a result of these early observations, a hypothesis was proposed that psoriasis is a disorder of abnormal keratinocyte proliferation mediated by T lymphocytes. It was further proposed that, in the initiation of psoriasis, activated CD4 cells produce cytokines which induce keratinocyte proliferation, and enhance angiogenesis and chemotaxis of lymphocytes into the dermis and epidermis. In the resolution of psoriasis, the activated CD8 cells produce cytokines, which may inhibit antigen-presenting cells, CD4 cells, keratinocyte proliferation and further chemotaxis of T cells into the epidermis. In chronic plaque psoriasis in which the psoriatic process is stable, there is a balance between the effects of the activated CD4 and CD8 cells. Thus, the activated CD4 cells are central to the hypothesis that T cells play a fundamental role in the development and maintenance of the psoriatic lesions.

Over the last 5 years, cytokines, produced by T cells, keratinocytes and other cell types found in the skin in psoriasis, have been identified and their function defined. Thus it is now becoming possible to propose a possible cytokine pathway for the initiation and maintenance of psoriasis. It is suggested that psoriasis is an antigen-dependent disease. When the antigen is present in the skin (dermis and epidermis), it is taken up by the antigen-presenting cells, which process the antigen, and the cell then becomes activated. These cells then release interleukin I (IL-I), which is chemotactic for T cells. Thus T cells are attracted to the antigen-presenting cells, and a number of these T cells will be antigen specific, that is have receptors which recognize the processed antigen. The processed antigen is then presented to the specific CD4 cell in association with the major histocompatability complex (MHC) class II antigen on the surface of the antigen presenting cell. The presentation of antigen, in association with the class II molecule, and IL-I produced by the antigen-presenting cell, are the two signals which will activate the CD4 cells. Once the CD4 cell becomes activated, it will produce a host of cytokines, including the interleukins IL-2, IL-3, IL-4, IL-6, IL-8 and interferon γ (IFN-γ). The functions of some of these cytokines are known. IL-2 is a T cell growth factor, so that the antigen-specific CD4 cells in the skin will proliferate and thus more CD4 cells are produced

which enhance the immune response. IL-2, IL-6 and IL-8 can stimulate keratinocytes to proliferate and to produce their own cytokines, and IFN-γ induces DR expression by cells including antigen-presenting cells (the Langerhans cells). In psoriasis there is an increase in the number of DR+ (activated) Langerhans cells which further enhances the psoriatic process. In addition, IFN-γ induces the expression of receptors for T cells in the endothelial cells of the capillaries, leading to a further influx of T cells. A number of the cytokines produced by the activated keratinocytes are similar to those produced by lymphocytes, that is IL-6 and IL-8. In addition, the activated keratinocytes produce IL-I and transforming growth factor-α (TGF-α). These three cytokines, IL-6, IL-8 and TGF-α, are capable of inducing keratinocyte proliferation and thus keratinocytes are capable of maintaining their own enhanced proliferation. The cytokines tumour necrosis factor-α (TNF-α), and IL-I produced by the Langerhans cells and keratinocytes, and IFN-γ, produced by activated CD4 cells, induce other changes which enhance this immune response. They increase the expression of intercellular adhesion molecule (ICAM), endothelial leukocyte adhesion molecule (ELAM), and vascular cell adhesion molecule (VCAM) in the endothelial cells of the capillaries, thus attracting more leukocytes, including T cells, into the skin. They also induce the expression of ICAM on the surface of cells in the dermis and epidermis, which increases the trafficking of T cells. Thus, this cytokine network can induce and maintain excessive keratinocyte proliferation characteristic of psoriasis, and is represented diagrammatically in Figure 6.

Resolution of psoriasis is not so well understood because the cytokines produced by CD8 cells and their action are still to be elucidated. However, they do produce cytokines which will inhibit the immune response. Their site of action may be on the antigen-presenting cell, CD4 cells, directly on the keratinocyte and the endothelial cell (Figure 7).

The cellular response of keratinocyte proliferation

and cytokine release in psoriasis is similar to that seen in normal wound healing after injury. Thus the question has to be asked as to why proliferation continues in psoriasis but not in wound healing. One of the possible explanations is that there is a failure of the keratinocyte in psoriasis to respond to the cytokines which normally inhibit keratinocyte proliferation. The cytokines which are known to inhibit cellular proliferation include IFN-γ, TNF-α, and TGF-β. It has already been shown that proliferation of psoriatic keratinocytes is not inhibited by IFN-γ to the same extent as that of normal keratinocytes. Thus, one of the defects in psoriatic skin may be failure to respond adequately to the normal homeostatic mechanisms of keratinocyte growth.

The above hypothesis depends on the presence of an antigen to trigger the psoriatic process. To date, the most likely antigen is a streptococcal one. As has already been mentioned, guttate psoriasis is often preceded by streptococcal infections. There is an increase in proliferative response by peripheral blood T lymphocytes to streptococcal antigens in both guttate and chronic plaque psoriasis. Finally, T cell clones that are reactive with streptococcal antigens have been isolated from guttate psoriasis lesions. Thus, there is now good evidence that streptococcal antigens may be involved in the initiation of psoriasis. There is also the possibility that streptococcal antigens may initiate psoriasis but, because of cross-reactivity with a self-antigen, psoriasis becomes an auto-immune process and self-perpetuating. Cross-reactivity has been demonstrated between certain keratins and streptococcal antigens, and homology has been demonstrated between keratin and a streptococcal protein (known as M6).

If the above hypothesis is correct, it has to be postulated at which stage, or stages, the genetic abnormality is operative. There are three possible sites (Figure 8). First, antigen presentation to T cells is dependent on the MHC class II molecules. It is known that DR7 is significantly increased in psoriasis, so that a possible structural difference of a class II molecule may be responsible for the presentation of the antigen. It is also possible that the genetic abnormality is expressed at the level of the T cell, which results in a different cytokine profile, compared to normal, being produced. This allows for increased keratinocyte proliferation. Thirdly, as has already been mentioned, the fault may be at the level of the keratinocyte in which there is an abnormal response to cytokines, whether it be stimulatory or inhibitory.

Finally, in support of the hypothesis that psoriasis is a T cell-mediated disease, is the observation that drugs, whose primary site of action is on CD4 cells, are effective in psoriasis. Thus, both cyclosporin and FK-506 are effective drugs in clearing psoriasis. It could be argued that, for the first time, a therapeutic agent was used for psoriasis based on scientific observation and not empiricism. The final conclusive evidence that activated CD4 is central to the pathogenesis of psoriasis is the demonstration that monoclonal antibodies to CD4 cells clear psoriasis.

The uninvolved skin

Although uninvolved skin in psoriasis looks normal, lesions may suddenly appear and involvement may occur at sites of injury to the skin. These observations, particularly the latter, imply that there may be an underlying abnormality in all the skin of psoriatic individuals. Certain abnormalities have now been described in the clinically uninvolved skin. There are increased numbers of T lymphocytes in the dermis, and both helper (CD4) and suppressor cells (CD8) are present, but it is predominantly the CD4 cells which are activated (DR+). There is an increase in the number of epidermal cells synthesizing DNA compared to normal, but it is less than that observed in lesional skin. Other abnormalities include enhanced polyamine synthesis, plasminogen activator activation, and increased levels of free arachidonic acid. These biochemical abnormalities are probably secondary to the increased cellular infiltrate. It is likely that the activated CD4 cells release cytokines which increase DNA synthesis of the epidermal cells and stimulate their metabolic activity. Thus the clinically uninvolved skin in psoriasis is in a state of readiness to develop psoriatic lesions under an appropriate stimulus. Once the activated CD4 cells move into the epidermis as a result of trauma or increased levels of antigen, then the psoriatic process will be initiated. The factors responsible for the influx of T lymphocytes into the dermis of psoriatic individuals are unknown at the present time. The influx may be related to increased levels and/or persistence of antigen in the skin.

Clinical features

Age of onset
Psoriasis may begin at any age, but it is rare under the age of 10 years. It is most likely to first appear between the ages of 15 and 30 years. In some 60% of patients, the disease will begin before the age of 30. The incidence of presentation then gradually falls with age, but psoriasis may first appear in the eighth and ninth decades. As a general rule, the earlier the age of onset the worse the prognosis.

Sex predilection
Psoriasis affects males and females equally.

Morphology
The classical lesion of psoriasis is a well demarcated raised red plaque with a white scaly surface (Figure 9). However, the colour of a psoriatic plaque depends on the thickness of the scale and whether it is adherent or loosely bound. The plaque colour may vary from red with a small amount of scale (Figure 10), to a white plaque with thick scale (Figures 11 and 12), to a greyish white colour (Figure 13), due to very thick adherent scale that is sometimes seen in untreated psoriasis.

A useful test to establish the diagnosis, if there is doubt, particularly when the lesion is a red non-scaly plaque, is to excoriate the lesion with a wooden spatula. If the lesion is psoriatic then the red plaque is turned into a white scaly one (Figure 14). This is due to the fact that the keratin in psoriasis is very loosely bound. If the keratin scales are lying flat, then visible light will pass through the keratin layers, and, when it reaches the dilated capillaries, the red part of the spectrum will be reflected, giving a red appearance in the plaque. However, when the loose keratin scales in psoriasis are disrupted by excoriation, the keratin lies at all angles to the surface and thus light (of all wave lengths) is reflected, giving a white appearance. A further useful sign if there is doubt about the diagnosis is to excoriate the lesion more vigorously and remove all the loosely bound keratin. A shiny surface (Figure 15) with capillary bleeding points (Figure 16) will then appear (Auspitz's sign).

Psoriasis tends to be a symmetrical eruption (Figures 17 and 18), and symmetry is a very helpful feature in establishing a diagnosis. Although unilateral psoriasis (Figure 19) may occur, it is the exception rather than the rule.

Sites and clinical patterns

Plaque psoriasis

This is the commonest form of psoriasis, and is the type seen in approximately 90% of patients. Plaque psoriasis is the usual form of presentation in adults. The lesions vary in number from one to several (Figures 19–23) and in size from 0.5 to 30 cm or more (Figures 20–25). If the disease is active, the plaques will merge to form large confluent areas of psoriasis (Figures 26–29). The commonest sites for psoriasis are the extensor surfaces of the elbows (Figure 17), knees (Figure 18) and scalp, but the skin on any part of the body may be involved, either with or without lesions elsewhere. Another common site is over the sacrum (Figure 30). The face is the site least likely to be involved. The disease presents as symmetrical well-demarcated red scaly plaques (Figures 17, 18, 22 and 23).

The extent of involvement may vary from less than 1 to 100% of the skin surface (when it is termed erythrodermic psoriasis). The course of plaque psoriasis varies. It may resolve spontaneously, even after many years, it may remain static, or it may progress with the enlargement of existing plaques and appearance of new ones. When plaque psoriasis clears, particularly when this occurs spontaneously, it tends to clear from the centre and the situation is reached when only the periphery of the plaque remains, giving rise to annular lesions (Figure 31). The latter type of lesion, therefore, tends to imply a good prognosis.

Temporary loss of pigment is not infrequent when psoriasis clears, giving rise to white macular areas (Figures 32 and 33).

Guttate psoriasis

This presents with the sudden appearance of small red papules, predominantly on the trunk (Figures 34–37). New lesions may continue to appear over the next month and may involve the limbs, face and scalp. The lesions tend to persist for 2–3 months, then resolve spontaneously. Thus, guttate psoriasis tends to be a self-limiting disorder. The lesions are approximately 0.5 cm and have little scale (Figures 34–36), although, if excoriated, white silvery scale will usually appear. Guttate psoriasis occurs more commonly in children, adolescents and young adults. Characteristically, it is preceded by a streptococcal sore throat. Some individuals have recurrent attacks of guttate psoriasis.

Very occasionally, guttate psoriasis lesions may enlarge (Figure 37) and persist; the disease then takes on the characteristics of chronic plaque disease (Figure 38).

Chronic plaque combined with guttate psoriasis

Patients who have established chronic plaque psoriasis sometimes develop typical guttate psoriasis. The guttate psoriasis lasts the usual 3 months, and the chronic plaque lesions may remain unaltered. On other occasions, the chronic plaque lesions enlarge when guttate psoriasis appears, and the disease generally becomes more active. In this situation, the enlarged plaques may not revert to their previous state when the guttate lesions resolve.

Koebner phenomenon

As previously described in the section on aetiology, the Koebner phenomenon is psoriasis appearing at the sites of trauma to the skin. The Koebner phenomenon does not occur in all patients. A patient may vary in time between being Koebner-positive and Koebner-negative. The nature of the injury is not specific. The clinical appearance of psoriasis in the Koebner phenomenon follows the site of injury. It may follow friction from tight clothing (Figure 39), a linear scratch (Figure 40), or occur at the site of an operation (Figure 41).

Erythrodermic psoriasis

This term is used when all the skin is involved in the psoriatic process (Figure 42). The skin is bright red, but the scaling is different from that seen in chronic plaque. There are no thick adherent white scales; instead there is superficial scaling. In erythrodermic psoriasis, the psoriatic process is at its most active, with increased proliferation and loss of maturation, and increased transit time; this in turn leads to abnormal keratin production, and keratin which is formed is loosely bound and quickly shed.

Patients with erythrodermic psoriasis lose excessive heat because of generalized vasodilatation of the cutaneous vessels. This may give rise to hypothermia. Thus patients with erythrodermic psoriasis are often found to be shivering, in an attempt to raise their body temperature. Oedema of the limbs develops because of the vasodilatation and loss of protein from the blood vessels into the tissues. High output cardiac failure and impaired hepatic and renal function may also occur in long-standing erythroderma.

Erythrodermic psoriasis usually develops from extensive chronic plaque or generalized pustular psoriasis, and implies that the disease is becoming more active.

Erythrodermic psoriasis is usually seen in young and middle-aged adults, but may occur at any age. There may be no exogenous trigger factors. However, known triggers include severe 'sunburn' (either from artificial ultraviolet light lamps or the sun), withdrawal of systemic steroids, irritation of the skin from coal tar and dithranol, and systemic infections. HIV infection may cause an exacerbation of existing psoriasis and this may become erythrodermic. Erythrodermic psoriasis is seen less commonly because treatments for extensive plaque psoriasis have improved over the last few years.

Erythrodermic psoriasis implies active disease and, therefore, usually a poor prognosis, particularly if there is no specific trigger. In the majority of patients, the disease reverts to extensive plaque disease with a tendency to further bouts of erythrodermic disease. If there is a specific trigger, then the prognosis is better and, provided the trigger can be avoided, there may be no further episodes of erythroderma.

Pustular psoriasis

There are two distinct entities to which the term pustular psoriasis refers. The first is generalized pustular psoriasis and the second, localized pustular psoriasis.

Generalized pustular psoriasis

This is an extremely rare form of psoriasis. It is usually preceded by other forms of the disease, i.e. chronic plaque, seborrhoeic (flexural), localized pustular psoriasis of the palms and soles, or acral psoriasis (see below). Generalized pustular psoriasis is usually seen in middle age and the sexes are equally affected.

The triggers which may be associated with generalized pustular psoriasis include withdrawal of systemic steroids, hypocalcaemia, infections (particularly upper respiratory tract) and local irritants, e.g. dithranol and ultraviolet light.

Four clinical patterns of generalized pustular psoriasis have been described, but, as is usual with clinical descriptive dermatology, there is some overlap between them.

The first is still sometimes referred to as the *Zumbusch pattern* after the person who first described it. It consists of a generalized eruption of sudden onset, with erythema and pustules (Figures 43 and 44). There is constitutional upset and a leukocytosis. The pustules are often superseded by sheets of scaling (Figure 45). The eruption lasts for a few weeks and then tends to revert to its previous state or it may transform to erythrodermic psoriasis (Figure 46). Subsequent episodes of generalized pustulation may follow.

An *annular* form of generalized pustular psoriasis may occur in which the pustules form in the periphery of red annular lesions. The annular form of the disease is probably a less severe form of the generalized Zumbusch pattern, and tends to be more persistent.

An *exanthematic* form of generalized pustular psoriasis tends to occur after a viral infection and consists of widespread pustules with generalized plaque psoriasis. However, unlike the Zumbusch pattern, there is no constitutional upset and the disorder tends not to recur.

A *localized* area of pustulation may occur in plaque psoriasis on the trunk and limbs (Figure 47) (distinct from the chronic form on the palms and soles). The localized area usually occurs after the application of an irritant, e.g. dithranol, or following the withdrawal of potent topical steroids. This localized form may simply be an extension of chronic plaque psoriasis but with an increase in the chemotactic factors for neutrophils.

At present, it is not known whether there are distinct pathogenic mechanisms in generalized pustular psoriasis, compared to chronic plaque disease, determined by genetic variation. Alternatively, the pustular phase is simply a more acute form of psoriasis with a greater release of chemotactic factors for neutrophils.

Localized pustular psoriasis

This term is used for a distinct clinical entity affecting the palms and soles (Figures 48 and 49). It is sometimes also referred to as persistent palmoplantar pustulosis. The disorder is usually seen in young and middle-aged adults and is more common in females.

The characteristic lesion is a well-defined area of redness and scaling with pustules. Frequently, reddish brown maculopapular lesions are also present (Figures 50–52) which are resolving pustules.

The discoid lesions may be solitary or multiple. They may remain the same size or occasionally enlarge and may coalesce and affect large areas of the palms and soles. Sometimes there is no definite edge to the affected area, and it is mainly a collection of pustules with associated scaling and erythema.

Localized pustular psoriasis may affect both palms and soles (in the same individual) or only the palms or soles. It is usually bilateral and symmetrical (Figure 49), but unilateral presentation may also occur. It is a very persistent condition; the lesions cleared in only one-third of patients in a 10-year follow-up study.

The relationship of localized pustular psoriasis to other forms of psoriasis is still unsettled. In favour of the localized palmar/plantar lesions being a form of psoriasis is the higher incidence of plaque psoriasis in patients with localized pustular psoriasis, compared to a control population. However, there is no reported increase of the HLA antigens, B13, B17, CW6 and DR7, in localized pustular psoriasis. There is also no increase in DNA synthesizing cells in the epidermis of the uninvolved skin, as occurs in the uninvolved skin of patients with plaque psoriasis.

Acral psoriasis

This variant of psoriasis begins on the fingers, and less frequently the toes (Figures 53 and 54), around the nails as small red scaly plaques. Pustules may be seen and there is associated nail dystrophy. Underlying bone changes may occur in the chronic form of disease. Proximal progression of the psoriasis tends to occur, and plaque lesions may develop at distinct sites. Eventual progression into generalized pustular psoriasis may follow.

Seborrhoeic psoriasis

In this form of psoriasis, the lesions tend to occur at the same sites as seborrhoeic eczema, i.e. the sides of the nose (Figure 55), around the mouth and eyes, the intertrigenous areas (Figures 56–58) and the centre of the chest. If there are no lesions elsewhere, then it may be difficult to distinguish this form of psoriasis from seborrhoeic eczema.

Childhood psoriasis

Chronic plaque psoriasis is rare in children, and guttate psoriasis is also not usually seen under the age of 5 years. One of the commonest forms of presentation in children is involvement of the genitalia (Figure 59) and perianal skin (Figure 60). This form of psoriasis tends to be persistent. Eventually, plaques of psoriasis tend to appear elsewhere on the trunk and limbs. Another form of presentation in children is of lesions appearing around the nails with an associated nail dystrophy (Figure 61). Psoriasis confined to the scalp may occur in children.

Napkin 'psoriasis'

This term is a misnomer as it implies that infants with this rash have psoriasis, and this is certainly not proven. The eruption usually begins between the ages of 3 and 6 months and first appears in the napkin area (although 'cradle cap' is usually present). The rash is a confluent red area confined to the napkin area (Figure 62). A few days later small red papules appear on the trunk (Figure 62) and may also involve the limbs. These papules have the typical white scales of psoriasis. The face may be involved with red scaly areas. Unlike psoriasis, the prognosis for this eruption in infancy is good and the rash responds well to treatment and tends to disappear after the age of 1 year.

Some reports have claimed that, although the rash in infancy disappears, it is a form of psoriasis and that there is a higher incidence of psoriasis in later life. However, this has been disputed in other reports. In addition, one study has shown that incidence of HLA antigens B13, B17 and B37 is no higher in infants with napkin 'psoriasis' compared to normal individuals. The word psoriasis should therefore not be used for this type of eruption; a more appropriate term is seborrhoeic eczema of infancy.

Linear psoriasis

This is a rare form of presentation. The psoriatic lesion presents as a straight line on limbs (Figure 63), or may be limited to a dermatome on the trunk. In adults, the aetiology of this form of the disease is unknown. In children it has been postulated as being due to an underlying naevus, which may predispose to the psoriatic process in susceptible individuals.

Psoriasis at specific sites
Scalp

The scalp is one of the commonest sites to develop psoriasis, and there may be no lesions elsewhere. Psoriasis of the scalp characteristically extends only to or just beyond the hair line (Figures 64 and 65). The commonest site of involvement of the scalp is behind the ears (Figures 65 and 66). Psoriasis of the scalp may present as discrete red raised scaly plaques, as found elsewhere on the trunk and limbs, or it may be diffuse scaling, or may present as very thick plaques of keratin with the scales growing along the hair shafts (Figure 67).

Hair loss with psoriasis of the scalp (Figure 68) is the exception rather than the rule. It does, however, occur with severe psoriasis, particularly the erythrodermic form of the disease. The alopecia presents as a diffuse thinning of the hair in the most severely affected areas, and may occur all over the scalp in erythrodermic psoriasis. The hair loss is reversible when the psoriasis clears, either with treatment or spontaneously.

Beard and pubic area
In patients with beards and in the pubic area (Figure 69), psoriasis may also be limited to the areas with hair. If the beard is shaved off, the psoriasis clears. No satisfactory explanation for this observation has been given.

Palms and soles
The palms and soles may be involved in plaque or guttate psoriasis. Occasionally, psoriasis (distinct from localized pustular psoriasis) may only affect the palms and/or soles. The appearance of psoriasis on the palms and soles tends to be different from the lesions elsewhere and this may give rise to diagnostic difficulty. The different clinical presentation is probably due to the different structure of the skin on the palms and soles. On the occasions when guttate psoriasis affects the palms and soles, it presents as hard reddish brown papules (Figure 70). There may or may not be some scale, but, if present, it is fairly adherent, unlike the lesions elsewhere on the trunk and limbs.

Plaque psoriasis may occur on the palms and soles with or without plaque lesions elsewhere. The palms and soles may have discrete lesions (Figure 71) or there may be confluent involvement affecting all the

plantar and palmar skin, including the digits (Figure 72). In the latter presentation, there is a sharp line of demarcation between the palmar and plantar involvement and the surrounding skin (Figure 73). Another form of palmar/plantar psoriasis presents as red fissured skin (Figures 74 and 75). There may be severe limitation of movement of the hand and/or foot with this type of lesion. The typical white flaky surface characteristic of psoriasis elsewhere may be absent (Figure 75). Occasionally, psoriasis on the palms and soles may present as so-called keratoderma. In this form there is very thick grey-white keratin. Fissuring is common and painful. Involvement of the soles leads to difficulty in walking, and on the palms there is severe limitation of normal function, so everyday tasks are difficult to perform, and manual occupations difficult to follow.

Flexures and intertrigenous areas
As mentioned above, psoriasis may predominantly involve the intertrigenous areas in so-called 'seborrhoeic psoriasis'. At other times, involvement of those sites may occur in plaque psoriasis (Figure 76). Psoriasis in an intertrigenous area is often limited to the area where the folds of skin are in actual contact; there is a sharp line of demarcation between the involved and uninvolved skin (Figures 56, 57 and 77). The psoriatic lesion may be raised or flat. The skin is red and has a shiny appearance and there is little or no scaling (Figures 56, 57, 76 and 77). This lack of scaling is due to the sweat in the intertrigenous area hydrating the keratin which inhibits scaling. If the opposing skin surfaces are kept apart for any length of time, superficial scaling with appear. In intertrigenous psoriasis, painful fissures may appear at the apex of the fold (Figures 77 and 78) . particularly the posterior natal cleft (Figure 78). The areas involved in intertrigenous psoriasis are the natal cleft, groins, axillae, submammary area, abdominal folds (in obese subjects) (Figure 77) and between the small toes.

Genitalia
The male genitalia are not an infrequent site for

psoriasis. It has been reported that between 2 and 5% of male patients have psoriasis on the penis. The commonest site of involvement is the proximal part of the glans. Small red well-demarcated plaques, varying from 0.5 to 2 cm are the typical lesions. The thick white scaling of ordinary plaque psoriasis is not usually present. In circumcised individuals, some superficial scaling may be seen but in the uncircumcised the patches have a shiny appearance. Plaques may also occur on the foreskin and shaft, but again thick white scales are not seen, and the appearance is that of a red patch with mild superficial scaling. Plaques and even confluent psoriasis may be present on the scrotum.

Involvement of the female genitalia is less common. The perivulval skin may be involved with confluent red well-demarcated lesions. There is only minimal scaling.

Mucous membranes

Involvement of the mucous membranes in psoriasis is very rare. Scaling of the lips is sometimes seen in the erythrodermic form. Involvement of the oral cavity in generalized pustular psoriasis occurs in a small percentage of these patients. There are discrete denuded areas with white slightly elevated edges. The appearances are similar to the geographical tongue, but in psoriasis the lesions are not confined to the dorsal surface of the tongue; they may also be seen on the buccal mucosae, ventral tongue and gingivae. The histology of the oral lesions is not that of psoriasis of the skin, and the pathogenesis is likely to be different.

Ocular lesions are rare in psoriasis, but blepharitis and keratitis have been reported; whether these are of a primary nature, or secondary to involvement of the skin of the eyelids is debatable.

Nails

Nail involvement in psoriasis is common. The incidence varies from 25 to 50% in reported studies. Involvement is more common in older individuals, extensive disease, and patients with psoriatic arthropathy. The lesions may be seen in the nail plate, due to involvement of the nail matrix, or the nail bed.

Nail pits   These are one of the commonest features of psoriasis and occur more frequently in the finger than the toe nails. Pits in the nail plate are approximately the size of a pinhead and may be solitary or multiple (Figures 79 and 80). They are thought to be due to small areas of psoriatic involvement in the nail matrix.

Terminal onycholysis   This is probably the second commonest feature of nail involvement and is usually seen in the finger and big toe nails. It is due to separation of the terminal nail plate from the nail bed. It presents as a whitish opaque area (Figures 80–82). Onycholysis may affect a solitary nail (Figure 81), a few, or all the nails (Figure 82). If several nails are affected, the involvement may be symmetrical. Onycholysis may only involve a small area under the nail or extend to 90% of the nail plate. If extensive, the nail may be lost, but another will regrow, and is also likely to show onycholysis.

Occasionally in onycholysis, bacteria grow under the nail plate and give rise to green (Figure 83) or black nails.

Oildrops   These are brownish translucent areas seen under the nail plate (Figure 84). They are due to small areas of psoriasis, giving rise to parakeratosis of the nail bed.

Subungual hyperkeratosis   This is most commonly seen in the toe nails (Figures 85 and 86). It is due to psoriasis of the nail bed with excessive production of keratin building up under the nail plate (Figure 85). It often leads to gross deformity of the nail, and destruction of the actual nail plate (Figures 86 and 87). This deformity may interfere with normal function of the fingers.

Thinning of the nail plate   This is due to total involvement of the nail matrix, resulting in a thin atrophic nail plate.

Nail haemorrhages   Small subungual, sometimes 'splinter', haemorrhages may be seen. These are due to trauma to the enlarged capillaries when psoriasis of the nail bed is present.

Differential diagnosis

The differential diagnosis will depend on the type of psoriasis and the site involved.

Chronic plaque psoriasis

Discoid eczema on the limbs in young adults presents as symmetrical discoid lesions, but in eczema there is not such a sharply defined edge between the involved and uninvolved skin. The surface of the lesion in eczema is less scaly and may be crusted.

Cutaneous T cell lymphoma (mycosis fungoides) may present as red discoid scaly lesions. However, in lymphoma the lesions are often asymmetrical, and the scaling is usually less. If there is a possibility of a lymphoma, a biopsy must be performed.

Bowen's disease usually presents as a red scaly plaque on the lower leg and occasionally mimics a solitary plaque of psoriasis. The scale in Bowen's disease is usually less than in psoriasis. A biopsy is necessary if there is doubt as to the correct diagnosis.

Pityriasis rubra pilaris is a rare disorder which presents with widespread red scaly plaques which may become confluent. Like psoriasis, there is a well-demarcated edge between involved and uninvolved skin. The disorder may be distinguished from psoriasis by the involvement of hair follicles. In pityriasis rubra pilaris, the follicles on the back of the fingers are frequently involved, giving rise to small red papules.

Guttate psoriasis

Pityriasis rosea affects a similar age group, and also occurs predominantly on the trunk. However, in pityriasis rosea the lesions are usually oval and have centripetal scaling. However, occasionally in pityriasis rosea the lesions are predominantly papular, and the diagnosis may then depend on the history and presence of a herald patch, and the type of scaling.

Secondary syphilis in its papular form is another eruption of sudden onset seen in young adults. However, in syphilis involvement of the palms, soles and face is common. If there is any doubt, serology tests for syphilis must be performed.

Occasionally endogenous *eczema* (particularly the seborrhoeic variety) may present as small red scaly papules and patches on the trunk. An eczematous eruption is usually less papular, but white silvery scales may be present in seborrhoeic eczema lesions.

The chronic form of *pityriasis lichenoides* presents as small red scaly papules. The distribution of pityriasis lichenoides differs from guttate psoriasis in that it is not predominantly on the trunk. The type of scale on the surface of the lesion is also different in pityriasis lichenoides, as it is more adherent.

Erythrodermic psoriasis

Eczema and *a cutaneous T cell lymphoma* may also

present as erythroderma. The appearance may be the same whatever the disease. A preceding history of eczema or psoriasis will be helpful in establishing the correct diagnosis, otherwise a biopsy will be necessary, particularly to diagnose the lymphoma.

Generalized pustular psoriasis

Subcorneal pustular dermatosis, if widespread, may have to be considered in the differential diagnosis, but in this disorder the pustules are often relatively large (i.e. 1 cm) and do not have the associated redness and scaling. Constitutional upset is not a feature of subcorneal pustular dermatosis.

Pemphigus foliaceous may have pustular lesions and be very extensive. The areas of involvement may also be red, scaly and slightly exudative.

Impetigo, if generalized, presents with widespread pustules, erythema and crusting. Swabs for bacteriology and biopsy will establish the diagnosis.

Migratory necrolytic erythema is a very rare disorder which may be generalized and have serpigenous lesions. The tongue is red and sore and the involvement is confluent, unlike the patchy lesions in psoriasis. Migratory necrolytic erythema is usually associated with a glucagonoma and so diabetes is usually present.

Widespread *candidal* infection in immunosuppressed patients may also present with widespread erythema and pustulation.

Localized pustular psoriasis

Infected eczema on the palms and soles may have a similar appearance to localized pustular psoriasis. Bacteriological tests may be needed to distinguish between the two conditions.

Fungal infection on the soles may be localized and produce vesicles and pustules. Therefore specimens

for mycology should always be taken if either condition is suspected.

Acral psoriasis

Herpes simplex, streptococcal and *candidal* infections have to be considered in the early stages when only one finger may be involved. The appropriate pathology tests should establish the diagnosis. Periungual eczema may also give a similar picture, but pustulation is unlikely unless secondary infection is present.

Seborrhoeic psoriasis

Seborrhoeic eczema is the obvious differential diagnosis. It may be extremely difficult to distinguish between the two conditions unless there are typical lesions of psoriasis elsewhere (including nail involvement). When involvement of the face occurs, psoriasis tends to be more scaly than eczema. HIV infection can cause a very florid seborrhoeic eczema eruption and also aggravate psoriasis. In the latter situation, it is not uncommon to see psoriasis flaring in a seborrhoeic 'distribution'. *Lupus erythematosus*, which affects the medial cheeks and nose, is not usually a scaly eruption and the other seborrhoeic sites are not involved.

Childhood psoriasis

As involvement of the genitalia, groins and perianal skin are common sites for psoriasis in children, the most likely differential diagnosis includes *seborrhoeic eczema* and *candidal infection*. Seborrhoeic eczema is uncommon in children (over the age of 2 years); lesions of psoriasis elsewhere and nail involvement help to establish the diagnosis. If there is involvement of the nails, then candidal and dermatophyte infections must be excluded by mycology tests.

Scalp psoriasis

Seborrhoeic eczema is the commonest disorder to mimic psoriasis of the scalp. If there are no lesions elsewhere, it may be impossible to distinguish between the two conditions. Psoriasis tends to give thicker lesions with more scale, and the lesions are more discrete, but these are not absolute distinguishing features. If hair loss is present *fungal infections* (particularly in children) will have to be excluded.

As a general rule, psoriatic hair loss does not give rise to scarring and thus can be distinguished from *discoid lupus erythematosus*.

Psoriasis of the palms and soles

Both the discrete discoid lesions, and the confluent involvement, of the palms and soles have to be distinguished from *chronic endogenous eczema*. In addition, both eczema and psoriasis may give rise to keratoderma (thick hyperkeratotic lesions) on the palms and soles. In confluent forms of psoriasis, there is a sharper line of demarcation between the involved and uninvolved skin compared to eczema. If the blisters are present or there is a history of vesiculation, this favours eczema.

Reiter's disease, which consists of urethritis, arthritis, ocular, skin and oral lesions, commonly presents with hyperkeratotic plaques on the palms and soles. The presence or history of urethritis, ocular and oral lesions should help to distinguish between psoriasis and Reiter's disease.

Flexural psoriasis

Seborrhoeic eczema (as discussed above, under seborrhoeic psoriasis) is the commonest disorder to be distinguished from psoriasis in intertrigenous areas.

Fungal infections and *erythrasma* may also be confined to flexural or intertrigenous areas. Erythrasma presents as sharply demarcated lesions in the groins and axillae, tends to have a reddish brown colour and fluoresces coral pink with ultraviolet light. Fungal infections in the axillae and submammary region are relatively rare, but common in the groins. The lesions tend to have a raised red scaly edge and eventually extend beyond the intertrigenous area. Secondary infection with *Candida albicans* in the intertrigenous areas presents with small satellite pustules surrounding the red plaque. Mycological and/or bacteriological tests should distinguish these infective problems from psoriasis.

Nails

The differential diagnosis depends on the type of nail lesions. Pitting of the nails without associated skin lesions around the nails is usually due to psoriasis. However, in *eczema* and *lichen planus*, pits have been described but there is skin involvement around the nails. Pits in nails have also been described in *alopecia areata* but hair loss is invariably present to elucidate the cause.

Onycholysis when it occurs without psoriatic skin lesions is sometimes referred to as idiopathic. It is more common on the finger nails, and in females. It is difficult to know whether idiopathic onycholysis is a separate entity or is due to underlying psoriasis. Onycholysis of the big toe nails may be due to trauma from foot wear. Onycholysis with subungual hyperkeratoses occurs in fungal infections and mycology tests will be necessary to distinguish between psoriasis and a fungal infection.

Subungual hyperkeratosis with dystrophy of the nail plate is more common in psoriasis of the toe nails than the finger nails, and has to be distinguished from *fungal infections* by mycology tests.

Green discoloration under the nail plates is seen with onycholysis, whether idiopathic or due to psoriasis. A greenish-brown discoloration may be seen, but usually at the sides of the nails in dystrophy secondary to chronic candidal paronychia. The chronic paronychia suggests the diagnosis of candida.

Pustulation around the nail seen in some forms of acral psoriasis may also occur in *chronic paronychia*, whether it be candidal or bacterial. Red scaly patches around the nail support the diagnosis of psoriasis, and the appropriate pathological tests should also be carried out.

Splinter haemorrhages under the nail, that may be seen in psoriasis, also occur in *fungal infections*, *minor trauma*, *connective tissue diseases* and *subacute bacterial endocarditis*. The history and other clinical features should help to establish the appropriate diagnosis.

Linear psoriasis

Linear psoriasis (which is very rare) has to be distinguished from *linear naevi*, *lichen striatus* (linear eczema) and *linear lichen planus*. The clinical appearance should suggest the diagnosis. If not, a biopsy should be performed.

Psoriatic arthropathy

An association between psoriasis and an arthritis was mentioned in the early part of the nineteenth century. However, there was no uniform agreement as to whether the arthropathy was part of the spectrum of rheumatoid arthritis or a separate entity. It is only in the past two or three decades that psoriatic arthropathy has been recognized as a separate disorder to rheumatoid arthritis. One of the problems in defining psoriatic arthropathy is whether it may exist without the skin lesions.

If this is accepted, then there appears to be significant overlap with ankylosing spondylitis and other spondarthritides. A working definition of psoriatic arthropathy would be 'an inflammatory arthritis, either peripheral or with spinal involvement, in association with psoriasis, and seronegative for the rheumatoid factor'.

Epidemiology

The incidence of arthropathy in patients with psoriasis has varied from 0.5 to 40% in different studies. This variation probably depends on the criteria used to establish the presence of an arthropathy, or missing the minimal skin involvement which may occur in some individuals. It would appear from the more careful studies that the incidence of an arthropathy in psoriasis is between 5 and 7%. The prevalence of arthritis in non-psoriatic dermatological patients has been reported as 0.7%.

Investigation of the incidence of psoriasis in patients with arthritis has shown a normal incidence for the seropositive, but an incidence four times the normal incidence in patients with seronegative arthritis, supporting the association between psoriasis and arthropathy. The overall incidence of psoriatic arthropathy in the general population has been estimated to be between 0.02 and 0.10%. The male : female sex ratio for psoriatic arthropathy has been shown to be 1:1.39, compared to 1:3 for rheumatoid arthritis.

Genetics

As with skin lesions, there is evidence to support a genetic mechanism in psoriatic arthropathy. Family studies have shown clustering, but no clear Mendelian pattern of inheritance has emerged. It appears that genetic transmission, as for the skin lesions, is based on multifactorial inheritance, with environmental factors playing an important part in triggering arthritis.

An increased incidence of HLA-B27 (95%) is now recognized in ankylosing spondylitis. This antigen has also been found to be raised in psoriatic arthritis if there is spinal involvement, the incidence being 80% for spinal involvement but 20% for peripheral arthritis. Other HLA antigens, A26, B38 and DR4, have been found to be raised in peripheral arthropathy.

Clinical features in peripheral arthropathy

There are five groups of psoriatic arthropathy which have been outlined.

(1) The most common presentation is mono- or asymmetrical oligoarthropathy. This usually affects the interphalangeal joints, either the distal or proximal (Figures 88 and 89).

(2) Exclusive involvement of the distal interphalangeal joints of the toes or fingers. Involvement of these joints is said to be characteristic of psoriatic arthropathy, and distinguishes it from rheumatoid arthritis, which does not affect these joints.

(3) The presentation which is indistinguishable from rheumatoid arthritis, but the psoriatic disease runs a more benign course.

(4) A severe mutilating arthritis, as seen in rheumatoid disease, but with involvement of the distal interphalangeal joints.

(5) A peripheral arthropathy associated with sacroiliitis and/or spondylitis.

The incidence of the common oligoarthropathy has been found to be 50% of the psoriatic arthropathies. The severe mutilating form and localization to the distal interphalangeal joints have an incidence of 8% each.

Of all psoriatic patients with arthropathy, 30% have spondylitis.

The peak age of onset for psoriatic arthropathy is between 35 and 45 years. The severe mutilating form usually begins earlier. The onset is acute in approximately 50% of patients. The skin and joint lesions do not usually commence at the same time, but nail dystrophy and joint involvement often appear together.

Spinal arthritis

There is now a recognized association between psoriasis and sacroiliitis and/or ankylosing spondylitis. The arthropathy may involve the sacroiliac joints and spine, together or separately. It is more common for both to be involved.

Relationship between skin lesions and arthropathy

The skin lesions appear first in the majority of patients, only 16% beginning with joint problems. In the latter group, those patients would be termed as having seronegative arthritis, until such time as they may develop the rash. It does appear that there may be a small group with classical features of psoriatic arthropathy, i.e. distal interphalangeal involvement, who do not go on to develop psoriasis.

There is a strong association between generalized pustular psoriasis and arthritis; 30% of these patients have an arthropathy. It has been found in some surveys that the more extensive the psoriasis, the more likely the arthropathy.

Relationship between nail involvement and arthropathy

There is a stronger association between joint involvement and nail abnormality than with skin lesions. It has been found that 85% of patients with arthropathy have nail involvement. The nail and joint problems often begin together. No particular one of the varying nail abnormalities is associated with the arthropathy.

Extra-articular features

These have a lower incidence than those of rheumatoid arthritis. Subcutaneous nodules and involvement of the lung, heart or blood vessels do not occur. Ocular involvement has been reported, mainly uveitis and conjunctivitis. Episcleritis is rare.

Ankylosing spondylitis and inflammatory bowel disease have an increased incidence in patients with psoriatic arthritis.

Treatment

In its mildest forms no specific treatment is necessary. The drug therapy for the arthritis is the same as that for rheumatoid arthritis. Non-steroidal anti-inflammatory drugs (NSAIDs) will control a large proportion of patients. In a small number of patients, the NSAIDs do appear to make the rash worse, but there is no way of predicting in which patient this may occur.

Other drugs which have been found to be helpful in severe disease are methotrexate, cyclosporin, azathioprine and gold salts. All have potential serious side-effects, and patients will have to be monitored closely. There are reports of improvement in the joints when the rash is treated with photochemotherapy (PUVA).

Drugs to be avoided are antimalarials and systemic steroids. The former have been reported to make the rash worse, and with the latter there may be a flare-up of the rash when the dose of steroids is reduced.

Surgical procedures as for rheumatoid arthritis should be considered if there is severe deformity.

Prognosis

The prognosis in psoriatic arthropathy appears to be better than in rheumatoid arthritis. There is generally less pain and disability. In a 10-year follow-up, one-third of the patients lost no time from work and 97% had less than 12 months absenteeism. Radiologically, there is little deterioration in the majority of patients. Most of the reported fatalities in psoriatic arthropathy have been attributable to the drugs employed, but there is a small risk of amyloidosis.

Treatment

The management of psoriasis depends on the individual who is the patient. Only a small proportion of patients suffering from psoriasis present with symptoms requiring treatment, e.g. irritation in a small proportion, painful fissures, where there is involvement of the palms and soles and in the intertrigenous areas, loss of mobility of the hands and feet with involvement at these sites, and systemic complications in erythrodermic and generalized pustular psoriasis. The main reason that patients seek treatment is because the disease is unsightly and therefore limits their social behaviour.

When individuals first present with psoriasis, it is essential that the nature of the disease is explained to them. It is important that patients are told that psoriasis is not contagious and, in the mild and moderate forms, there are no serious complications. It should also be stressed that, apart from a genetic factor, the cause of the disease is not fully understood. The natural history should be explained and it must be emphasized that at present doctors cannot cure the disease, or even modify the course of the illness. Current treatments do not affect disease activity. If the disease is active, then relapse will occur as soon as treatment is discontinued whatever therapy is used. The chance of remissions and their length do not depend on treatment. However, it is also important that patients are told that it is always possible to clear psoriasis with treatment currently available.

Many patients may choose not to treat their psoriasis when they realize the limitations of current therapeutic agents and are told of the benign nature of their disease. Other patients are unable to tolerate even minimal disease and demand treatment.

Most of the therapeutic agents used to treat psoriasis are based on empiricism or chance observations. It is only over the last few years that new drugs are being tried based on scientific observation. The current treatments can be divided into topical agents, those based on ultraviolet light, and systemic drugs.

Topical drugs
There are four drugs used topically, corticosteroids, coal tar, dithranol and the vitamin D analogue, calcipotriol.

Topical corticosteroids
There is a good correlation between the potency of the steroid and its antipsoriatic action. Thus the stronger the steroid the better it is at clearing psoriasis. Because of the wide variations in the potency of topical steroids, it is standard practice to divide them into four groups depending on their strength. The potency of a topical steroid is determined by biological assay (usually fibroblast inhibition or vasoconstriction). Hydrocortisone, which is the weakest topical steroid, is used as the standard with which to compare others.

Hydrocortisone (group I, a weak steroid) is designated to have 1 unit of steroid activity, moderate strength steroids (group II) 25 units, strong steroid 100 units (group III) and very strong, 600 units (group IV). Thus the range of steroid activity in those currently available, is 1–600 units. It is important when prescribing topical steroids that the physician knows to which group the steroid belongs. Table I groups the majority of topical steroids in current use, depending on their potency.

Topical steroids can be applied as a lotion for scalp lesions, a cream for facial and intertrigenous areas, and an ointment for lesions on the trunk and limbs.

Advantages   The main advantage of topical steroids is that they are pleasant to use. Group III and IV steroids are moderately effective in clearing chronic plaque psoriasis. Group II and III steroids can clear facial and intertrigenous psoriasis. Group III and IV

Table I   Topical corticosteroids

	Generic name	*Trade name (UK)*	*Trade name (USA)*
Group I (weak)	Hydrocortisone (0.5%, 1% and 2.5%)	Efcortelan Hydrocortistab Hydrocortisyl Hydrocortone	Cort-Dome Cortril Dermacort Heb-Cort Hytone
	Alclometasone dipropionate (0.05%)	Modrasone	Alcovate
Group II (intermediate strength)	Clobetasone butyrate (0.05%) Hydrocortisone butyrate (0.1%) Flurandrenolone (0.0125%) Flurandrenolone acetonide (0.025%) Fluocortolone pivalate (0.1%) + fluocortolone hexanoate (0.1%)	Eumovate Locoid Haelan Ultradil	 Cordran
Group III (strong)	Betamethasone valerate (0.1%) Betamethasone (0.2%) Fluocinolone acetonide (0.025%) Halcinonide (0.1%) Fluocinonide (0.05%) Beclomethasone dipropionate (0.025%) Fluclorolone acetonide (0.025%) Triamcinolone acetonide (0.1%) Fluocortolone pivalate (0.25%) + fluocortolone hexanoate (0.25%) Flumethasone pivalate (0.03%) Betamethasone dipropionate (0.05%) Diflucortolone valerate (0.1%)	Betnovate Synalar Halciderm Metosyn Propaderm Topilar Adcortyl Ledercort Ultralanum Diprosone Nerisone	Valisone Celestone Synalar Fluonid Halog Lidex — — Aristocort Locorten Diprolene
Group IV (very strong)	Clobetasol propionate (0.05%) Fluocinolone acetonide (0.2%) Diflucortolone valerate (0.3%)	Dermovate Nerisone forte	Temovate Synalar HP

steroids in alcoholic solution are able to improve or sometimes clear lesions of the scalp.

Disadvantages   One of the main disadvantages of topical steroids is that tachyphylaxis occurs when they are used for psoriasis. This means that the topical steroid will eventually lose its antipsoriatic effect. To maintain the clinical efficacy, the strength of the steroid will have to be increased and this increases the chance and incidence of side-effects. There is a limit to the strength of topical steroid available and, when this is reached, then topical steroids are no longer effective.

Side-effects   These are proportional to the strength of steroid and duration of use. In addition, side-effects are more commonly seen in intertrigenous areas because of the greater absorption of the drug at these sites, due to the moist environment, and the face where the skin is relatively thin. The local side-effects are due to collagen atrophy and inhibition of fibroblasts, and clinically these present as thin skin (Figure 90), telangiectasia (Figure 91), striae (Figure 92) and spontaneous bruising and purpura (Figure 93). Suppression of the pituitary adrenal axis and possibly cushingoid features only occur with group IV (and very occasionally group III) steroids. Topical steroids have to be used over long periods to produce these side-effects. As a general rule, 50 g of a group IV and 300 g of a group III steroid will have to be applied in a week to cause suppression of the pituitary adrenal axis.

Very occasionally, there can be a flare-up of the psoriasis when the topical steroid treatment is discontinued. This is usually only seen after the use of group IV steroids. The plaque may become pustular and enlarge. This rebound phenomenon may settle by itself; if not, weaker topical steroids (group II or III) may help. If the lesions are numerous and become more extensive, then one of the systemic drugs may have to be used.

In the past, topical steroids were used under polythene occlusion dressings to increase their efficacy. These dressings should not be used as they will also increase the incidence and severity of side-effects.

Indications   Group II and III topical steroids (in a cream base) are indicated for intertrigenous and facial psoriasis, as other topical drugs cannot be used at these sites.

Group III and IV steroids in an alcoholic lotion may be used on the scalp, if other preparations are not effective or tolerated.

Group III and IV steroids may be used for plaque psoriasis on the trunk and limbs. They should only be used as short courses, i.e. 2–3 weeks, and then stopped. If used for long periods, tachyphylaxis will occur and over long periods thinning of the surrounding skin may ensue.

Group II and III steroids are sometimes helpful in enhancing the resolution of guttate psoriasis.

Efficacy   Topical steroids are moderately effective in the treatment of psoriasis.

Coal tar preparations

Coal tar preparations are the oldest substances still employed in the treatment of psoriasis, although they are being used less frequently. Crude coal tar is a mixture of approximately 10 000 compounds. Purification of the crude coal tar by distillation produces other mixtures which are pleasanter to use, but less efficacious. The mechanism of action of coal tar in psoriasis is unknown.

Preparations   Crude coal tar is usually made up in an ointment base or as a paste. The concentration is usually 5–10%. Crude coal tar is often combined with salicylic acid 2–5%, which by its keratolytic action leads to better absorption of the coal tar.

Crude coal tar is only used to treat chronic plaque psoriasis and is usually combined with ultraviolet light.

Liquid coal tar is used in a variety of preparations for psoriasis. It is more acceptable to patients than crude coal tar. It is combined with keratolytics for use as a scalp preparation (10% liquid coal tar, 5% salicylic acid, 5% sulphur, 40% coconut oil, 40% emulsifying ointment). This particular preparation is usually applied at night and shampooed out the next morning. Liquid coal tar is frequently added to the bath water, either undiluted or in proprietary preparations. It may also be added to emulsifying ointment (15–20% of liquid coal tar) and applied to the skin before the patients gets into the bath.

Purified coal tar is added to shampoos, but has very little effect on scalp psoriasis.

Purified coal tar preparations are also used in cream and ointment bases for chronic plaque psoriasis, but, although cosmetically acceptable to the patient, their efficacy is poor.

Advantages   Coal tar products are relatively safe and have very few side-effects.

Disadvantages   Occasionally patients become sensitive to the coal tar and develop allergic reactions. A folliculitis may occur after the use of coal tar. The main disadvantage is the smell of crude coal tar. It is also unpleasant to use as it stains the clothes and bed clothes and the preparation has to be applied under tube gauze dressings. This makes it difficult to use as an outpatient unless the patient attends a special day centre, which has its own drawback in that it is time consuming, the patient having to attend hospital each day.

Efficacy   This is relatively low compared to other drugs available for the treatment of psoriasis. The purified coal tar products are less efficacious than the unpurified coal tar preparations.

Indications   For plaque psoriasis use crude coal tar as a paste or ointment, or purified coal tar in a cream or ointment base. Liquid coal tar can be added to the bath water or emulsifying ointment for baths. For scalp psoriasis use liquid coal tar combined with keratolytics, and coal tar shampoos.

Contraindications   Coal tar products should not be used in the acute forms of psoriasis, i.e. guttate, erythrodermic or pustular psoriasis, as they may aggravate these conditions.

Dithranol
Dithranol, 1,8-dihydroxy-9-anthrone is a naturally occurring substance found in the bark of the aroroba tree in South America. It can also be synthesized from anthrone. Its antipsoriatic action was noted over 100 years ago, when an extract of aroroba bark was used to treat psoriasis. The mechanism of action of dithranol in the treatment of psoriasis is still speculative.

Preparations   Dithranol is made up in either a cream, ointment or paste. It is also available in a proprietary preparation of grease sticks. The advantage of using dithranol in a paste is that it is less likely to spread on to the surrounding skin. The disadvantage of using a paste is that it is difficult to remove.

There are two ways of using dithranol, either as an application over a 24-hour period, or as an application for only 15–30 minutes (short-contact dithranol). When used for 24 hours it is advisable to start with a concentration of 0.1%; if there is no burning or soreness then the concentration is gradually increased, usually every 3–4 days, to a maximum of 1.0%. It usually takes 3–4 weeks to clear psoriasis with dithranol. When used as a short-contact treatment, the initial concentration of dithranol is usually 2% and this may be increased to a maximum of 4%. The time taken to clear psoriasis with short-contact treatment is approximately the same as for the 24-hour treatment.

Short-contact treatment is usually given on an outpatient basis. It is imperative that the patient complies with the instructions, otherwise side-effects will occur. Short-contact treatment should not be recommended if compliance is in doubt.

Advantages   Dithranol is probably the most effective topical antipsoriatic preparation currently available.

Disadvantages   There are two main problems with dithranol treatment. First, dithranol stains the skin surrounding psoriatic plaques (Figure 94), the clothes, bed clothes, furniture and the bath a purple-brown colour. Thus patients must be warned about this problem and dithranol must be used under tube gauze dressings. Patients should wear old pyjamas when the drug is applied for 24 hours. When used for short-contact therapy, patients must wear old pyjamas or clothes that they do not mind staining. The staining of the skin lasts up to 2 weeks after the dithranol is discontinued. It is difficult to remove the stains from clothing, bed clothes and furniture. The stains can be removed from the bath with either potassium permanganate or the detergent Teepol. The second problem with dithranol is that it causes an inflammatory reaction on the surrounding non-lesional skin. In its mildest form it is simply erythema; in its more severe forms it produces blisters (Figure 95) and erosions. This inflammatory reaction is accompanied by a burning sensation. If it is severe, the dithranol treatment has to be discontinued. Because of the inflammatory reaction to dithranol on non-lesional skin, dithranol should not be used in the intertrigenous areas, on the face or near mucous membranes. If dithranol gets in the eyes, it can cause a severe inflammatory reaction with subsequent scarring of the conjunctivae.

Efficacy   This is high, if the dithranol can be tolerated.

Indications   Dithranol should only be used for chronic plaque psoriasis on the limbs and trunk.

Contraindications   It should not be used for guttate, erythrodermic or pustular psoriasis.

Calcipotriol

This is a relatively new topical treatment for psoriasis. Calcipotriol is an analogue of vitamin D3; it has the same antipsoriatic action as vitamin D3, but only 10% of the effect on calcium metabolism. Topical vitamin D was first used for psoriasis after the observation that patients, who also had psoriasis, taking vitamin D for osteoporosis, had improvement of their skin disorder. Topical vitamin D preparations were then shown to be effective but only in a concentration which had an effect on calcium metabolism.

There are two postulated mechanisms for the beneficial effect of calcipotriol in psoriasis. First, vitamin D enhances differentiation of epithelial cells, and in psoriasis there is lack of differentiation of keratinocytes. Second, vitamin D is said to affect immune responses by inhibiting T helper (CD4) lymphocytes.

Preparation   There is currently only one topical preparation of calcipotriol and this is a an ointment, with a concentration of 0.005%.

Advantages   Like topical steroids, calcipotriol cream is a pleasant preparation to use.

Disadvantages   To date, the only reported side-effects are irritation and an irritant eczematous rash, particularly on the face. Therefore, calcipotriol should only be used on the limbs and trunk, and, if applied with a finger, the hands must be washed after use of the cream.

Calcipotriol has only been in use for a relatively short period and thus the possible long-term effect on calcium metabolism has to be remembered.

Efficacy   There are mixed reports on the antipsoriatic effect of calcipotriol. Its efficacy appears to be moderate, and similar to a group III steroid.

Indications   Calcipotriol is only indicated in chronic plaque psoriasis on the trunk and limbs.

Ultraviolet light

It has been known for over 100 years that sunlight benefits psoriasis, and ultraviolet light has been used for treatment for 70 years. Ultraviolet light from artificial sources may be used by itself (phototherapy) or combined with drugs (photochemotherapy). Ultraviolet light can be divided into short wave (UVC 250–290 nm), middle wave (UVB 290–320 nm) and long wave (UVA 320–400 nm). UVC does not penetrate the earth's atmosphere, and benefit from sunlight is therefore from the UVB and UVA. The erythema and 'sunburn' effect of ultraviolet light is produced mainly by UVB. It requires a 1000 times greater dose for UVA to produce a similar effect. However, UVA intensity at the solar zenith is 100 times greater than UVB, and persists for much more of the day, so its effects in sunlight are not minimal. The main limiting factor of using ultraviolet light as a treatment for psoriasis is the 'sunburn' reaction. The paler the skin the more likely the patients are to 'burn'. This limits the amount of light they can receive, meaning the treatment is less effective. Patients can be divided into groups depending on their skin colour, their ability to withstand the burning effect of ultraviolet light and their ability to tan. This classification is helpful in predicting the suitability of a particular patient for ultraviolet light treatment:

Group 1 – always burn, never tan
Group 2 – always burn, sometimes tan
Group 3 – sometimes burn, always tan
Group 4 – never burn, always tan
Group 5 – yellow-brown races
Group 6 – blacks

Phototherapy

This is carried out with UVB-emitting lamps. The apparatus is now so constructed that the whole body can be treated simultaneously. It consists of a cabinet, somewhat like a telephone kiosk, with fluorescent tubes on the walls. The initial dose will depend on the skin type, and may be gradually increased providing there is no burning of the skin. Treatment is usually carried out 3–4 times per week. Patients have to wear protective goggles during treatment to screen out the UVB from their eyes.

Advantages   The main advantage of UVB treatment is that no topical ointments, creams or oral medication are necessary. Patients with longstanding psoriasis find it a relief not to have to apply messy creams and ointments.

Disadvantages   One of the principal disadvantages is that patients have to attend hospital on a regular basis for their treatment. If they do not live near the hospital, then it becomes a very time-consuming exercise or even an impossibility. UVB lamps for home use are available, but they are expensive.

With UVB irradiation alone, the clinical improvement is slow and it may take 6–8 weeks to clear or achieve significant improvement of psoriasis. Maintenance treatment will probably be required for severe or active disease.

The only immediate potential side-effect is possible burning of the skin, if the dose is too high for that particular individual.

The long-term hazard of UVB treatment is its possible carcinogenic effect. There is some circumstantial evidence that basal and squamous cell carcinomas are due to chronic exposure to ultraviolet light, whilst melanoma may be induced by an acute sunburn reaction. Thus care must be taken not to burn patients. Possibly, the treatment should not be continued indefinitely.

Efficacy UVB alone is only of moderate efficacy, compared to photochemotherapy and is one of the slowest forms of treatments to produce clearance.

Indications   Phototherapy is indicated for chronic plaque psoriasis not responsive to topical measures. It is not effective for scalp or intertrigenous psoriasis because the UVB rays do not reach these sites. Phototherapy is sometimes used for guttate psoriasis to speed resolution.

Contraindications UVB should not be used for erythrodermic or generalized pustular psoriasis.

Photochemotherapy (PUVA)

This treatment is based on the photosensitizing chemicals, psoralens. These occur naturally in plants but can also be synthesized. Psoralens exert their photosensitizing effect by absorbing light and then releasing this energy within the skin to exert biological effects. Psoralens also have the ability to combine with DNA in the presence of ultraviolet light. This was thought to be the basis of its action in psoriasis, as it would lead to inhibition of mitoses of the epidermal cells and hence proliferation. However, ultraviolet light also inhibits the function of antigen-presenting cells and lymphocytes and this effect is increased in the presence of psoralens.

The basis for PUVA (psoralens + UVA) treatment was the observation that UVA is 1000 times less likely to induce erythema and burning of the skin compared to UVB. It was suggested that, if only UVA was used, the psoralens would still exert their antiproliferative action, and yet 'burning' would be avoided. In practice, the combination of psoralens and UVA has proved to be a highly effective treatment for psoriasis.

Patients have to take the psoralens 2 hours before the UVA irradiation. The dose depends on body weight. The psoralen preparation usually used is 8-methoxy-psoralen. The dose is 20 mg if the body weight is under 50 kg, 30 mg if 51–65 kg, 40 mg if 66–80 kg, and 50 mg if over 80 kg. The treatment is carried out 3–4 times per week. The amount of UVA given initially depends on the skin type, and patients can be tested before treatment to determine the appropriate starting dose. The amount of UVA (measured in joules) is gradually increased to achieve satisfactory clearance of the psoriasis without inducing side-effects. Patients have to wear protective spectacles

after taking the psoralen tablets and for at least the next 6 hours, as the eyes will be more sensitive to natural ultraviolet light and UVA from fluorescent lamps.

There are various machines for giving UVA treatment depending on the site of the psoriasis. There are machines designed to treat the whole body, or only hands or feet or scalp. The lamps used emit only UVA and visible light.

Advantages PUVA therapy has the same advantages as phototherapy with UVB, but it is more effective and quicker to achieve clearance than UVB alone.

Disadvantages Regarding the immediate side-effects, one of the main problems with PUVA is that the psoralens may cause nausea. This can be lessened to some extent by taking the drugs with food, or giving metoclopramide with the psoralens. Erythema and burning may occur, and if so the dose of UVA must be decreased. Pruritus is not an uncommon symptom, and pain may also be experienced. The pain and pruritus may be transitory, or prolonged, i.e. for many weeks, even though the treatment is discontinued. The cause of these symptoms is unknown but it has been suggested that it may be due to inflammation and damage to the nerve endings in the skin. A side-effect of PUVA, but one to which the patients do not usually object, is tanning.

The long-term side-effects include premature ageing of the skin. If PUVA is continued as maintenance therapy or patients have repeated courses, then changes due to photoageing may be seen. These changes will depend on the amount of joules and the skin type. Lentigos are the commonest feature (Figure 96), but thinning and dryness of the skin also occur. Damage to the elastic tissue leads eventually to wrinkling.

There is a definite increase in squamous cell carcinoma in patients who have received long-term

PUVA. There is good correlation between the incidence of squamous cell carcinoma and the total dose of PUVA. The male genitalia appear to be a particular site at risk and this area should therefore be covered when patients are having total body PUVA. To date, there appears to be no significant increase in basal cell carcinomas or melanoma (PUVA started 16 years ago, and an increase in melanoma may still occur).

PUVA therapy has been reported to cause immunosuppression not only of the skin but also of a general nature. This has been attributed to the large proportion of lymphocytes that perfuse the skin whilst patients are receiving treatment. To date, however, there are no reports of disorders associated with general immunosuppression.

Females who are pregnant or are contemplating pregnancy should not receive PUVA.

As with phototherapy, PUVA is not effective for scalp or intertrigenous psoriasis, as the UVA does not reach these areas.

Efficacy PUVA is a very effective treatment for psoriasis, and approximately 95% of patients who can tolerate the treatment will have good results. Nausea and pruritus are the main limiting factors.

Indications PUVA is indicated for chronic plaque disease which is extensive or has failed to respond to topical treatment. It is also effective for localized pustular psoriasis of the palms and soles. It is effective in guttate psoriasis, but, because this condition is of short duration, PUVA is not usually indicated.

Contraindications PUVA, as a general rule, should not be used for erythrodermic or pustular psoriasis.

Bath photochemotherapy

Instead of taking psoralens by mouth, they can be used topically to achieve the same effect. However, applying the psoralen solution by a brush has led to varying concentrations on the skin. This may lead to unwanted side-effects and a non-uniform clinical response. To surmount this problem, the psoralen is added to bath water and the patient takes a bath prior to the UVA irradiation. The advantage of 'bath PUVA' is that the common side-effect of nausea following oral psoralens is circumvented. The main disadvantage of bath PUVA is that a bath has to be provided at the PUVA treatment centre, so the time patients have to spend at the hospital is considerably lengthened.

Climatic therapy

Many patients know that going to a sunny climate improves their psoriasis, but there are a small proportion of patients who find that their psoriasis may actually deteriorate in the sun. For those whose psoriasis improves, the nearer the equator the more potent the effects of the sunlight. Patients should be warned not to over-expose themselves in the first few days, as sunburn may actually progress to psoriasis (the Koebner phenomenon). It usually takes 4 weeks to clear psoriasis in an appropriate climate.

As already mentioned, one of the problems of self-treatment in the sunnier parts of the world is sunburn. This problem is overcome by going to the Dead Sea. This curious result is due to the unique geographical features of the Dead Sea. It is the deepest place on the Earth's surface and is surrounded by mountains. The sea evaporates and forms an aerosol which stays in the atmosphere above the sea and surrounding beaches. This aerosol screens out the majority of the UVB rays but not the UVA. This mixture of ultraviolet light at the earth's surface is sufficient to clear psoriasis but prevent sunburn. Thus patients can stay on the shores of the Dead Sea all day without risk of sunburn. It is also claimed that the chemicals in the Dead Sea speed the resolution of psoriasis. There is no doubt that the Dead Sea is more effective than other parts of the world in clearing psoriasis, but it still takes 4 weeks for this to happen. The only disadvantages of this treatment are time and expense.

Oral therapy

There are three drugs (methotrexate, etretinate, cyclosporin) in current use for systemic treatment of psoriasis. They are limited to severe disease as they all have potential serious side-effects. The drug chosen as the first line of systemic treatment is the personal choice of the physician.

Methotrexate

Methotrexate is a folic acid antagonist which has been used for psoriasis for the last 40 years. The beneficial effect on psoriasis was a chance observation when these drugs were being used for rheumatoid arthritis for a supposed anti-inflammatory effect. A number of patients with psoriatic arthritis were also included in the study, and it was noted that the psoriatic skin lesions cleared.

Methotrexate is given weekly. A test dose of 5.0 mg should be given and if there are no untoward side-effects, the dose can be increased. The dose to clear psoriasis varies between patients but is usually 10–30 mg weekly. Very occasionally, a higher dose may be necessary. The dose for a particular patient has to be found by altering the dose according to the clinical response.

Prior to initiating methotrexate, patients must have a full blood count, liver function tests, serum creatinine, urine analysis, and chest X-ray. Patients with abnormal liver or renal function should probably not be given methotrexate. Whether a liver biopsy is performed prior to initiating methotrexate is a matter of choice for the physician. Routine monitoring of full blood count and liver function are mandatory. If patients are to take methotrexate for long-term maintenance therapy, then a liver biopsy should probably be performed every 2–3 years, or sooner if there are indications. However, liver biopsy is not without morbidity and even mortality, and therefore the decision to perform a liver biopsy has to be taken at an individual level, and not necessarily carried out routinely.

Advantages Methotrexate is a highly effective drug in clearing psoriasis and maintaining the improvement.

Disadvantages Regarding the immediate side-effects, some patients experience nausea and lethargy for 24–48 hours after taking methotrexate. Oral and gastrointestinal ulceration and suppression of the bone marrow are the main immediate side-effects. Some patients appear to be sensitive to these side-effects and this is the reason for giving a small test dose prior to initiating treatment to clear psoriasis. Once the patient is established on a maintenance dose, the risk of ulceration of the alimentary tract and bone marrow suppression recedes.

The main long-term side-effect is damage to the liver. Methotrexate is hepatotoxic and there may be a slight rise in liver enzymes in the first few days after taking the drug. However, this hepatoxicity may lead to fibrosis and eventually cirrhosis. The risk of serious liver damage is related to the cumulative dose and duration of treatment. Thus the longer the treatment is continued, the greater the indication for liver biopsy to assess liver histology. It is important that, if changes are seen on biopsy, they be assessed by a person experienced with methotrexate hepatotoxicity.

Efficacy Methotrexate is very effective in clearing psoriasis.

Indications Methotrexate is indicated for severe plaque psoriasis unresponsive to topical measures and ultraviolet light treatments, and erythrodermic and generalized pustular psoriasis.

Contraindications Methotrexate is contraindicated in pregnancy, severe impairment of hepatic or renal function, and if patients are receiving drugs which interact with methotrexate.

Etretinate

Etretinate is a retinoid. These are analogues of vitamin

A and were developed primarily as anti-cancer agents. The observation, that vitamin A deficiency is associated with follicular hyperkeratoses, dryness of the lips and general dryness of the skin, led to the suggestion that some of the analogues of vitamin A may improve disorders associated with abnormal keratinization.

Of the vitamin A analogues available, etretinate has been found to be helpful in psoriasis. The dose is 0.5–1.0 mg/kg per day. When used as the sole treatment for plaque psoriasis, it may take up to 3 or 4 months before there is significant improvement. However, the beneficial effect on generalized pustular psoriasis is apparent within days.

Advantage   As with other oral treatments, the simplicity of use is of considerable benefit to the patient.

Disadvantages   Probably the most important side-effect of all retinoids is that they are teratogenic. Unfortunately, etretinate is not totally cleared from the body for 2 years after discontinuing the drug. Therefore, as a general.rule, women of child-bearing age should not receive etretinate for psoriasis.

Immediate side-effects   After approximately 2 weeks, patients develop dryness and peeling of the lips. In the more severe forms of cheilitis, there may be fissuring and secondary infection. Other mucous membranes may also be affected, particularly the nasal mucosa leading to epistaxis. Conjunctivitis is a more rare complication. The skin may become red and scaly and this is more common on the face. Another rare complication is swelling and redness of the nail folds, mimicking paronychia. Scaling of the scalp and diffuse thinning of the hair may also occur. All the side-effects are reversible when the etretinate is discontinued.

Long-term side-effects   A rise in serum lipids occurs in nearly half of the patients taking long-term etretinate. This increase is reversible when the drug is discontinued. Hepatotoxicity is a rare complication. Extra-osseous ossification may occur around joints. The true incidence of this complication is not known because radiographs are not routinely taken during therapy.

Efficacy   The beneficial effect of etretinate is variable between patients. A major drawback is that it is slower than methotrexate and cyclosporin in clearing psoriasis.

Indications   Etretinate is indicated for severe plaque psoriasis unresponsive to topical measures and ultraviolet light treatments, and generalized pustular psoriasis.

Contraindications   Etretinate is contraindicated in hyperlipidaemia and impaired liver function, and should not be used by pregnant women, and ideally women of child-bearing age.

Cyclosporin

Cyclosporin has been used for psoriasis for the last 5 years. It was used intentionally because of the known action of cyclosporin in inhibiting activated CD4 (T helper) lymphocytes, which are central to the pathogenesis of psoriasis.

The initial dose of cyclosporin for psoriasis should be 3 mg/kg per day. If there is no significant improvement after 2 weeks, the dose may be increased to 4 mg/kg per day. If there is no improvement after a further 2 weeks, the dose may be increased to 5 mg/kg per day. However, this latter dose should not be exceeded because there is an increased risk of side-effects. A small proportion of patients are able to control their psoriasis with a daily dose of 2 mg/kg. The dose may vary from time to time in an individual depending on the activity of the disease.

Prior to treatment with cyclosporin, it is mandatory to ensure that patients have normal renal function. Serum creatinine and urine analysis may not be sensitive enough to identify early renal damage, and therefore, ideally, the glomerular filtration rate should be determined before initiating treatment. A full blood count and liver function tests should also be taken before starting treatment. The blood pressure must also be taken before beginning treatment.

During treatment, regular monitoring (approximately every 4–6 weeks) of blood pressure, serum creatinine and liver function is necessary. If long-term treatment is undertaken, then the glomerular filtration rate should be determined annually. A small decrease of the glomerular filtration rate is to be expected but, if it is greater than 35%, then cyclosporin should probably be discontinued. A rise in serum creatinine greater than 30% of the baseline value also implies significant impairment of renal function and it is advisable to try to control the psoriasis with a lower dose if possible. If the serum creatinine rises to more than 50% of the baseline value, then cyclosporin should be discontinued.

Because there is a relatively good correlation between renal function (as measured by the glomerular filtration rate) and renal biopsy findings during long-term cyclosporin treatment, it is probably not necessary to perform routine renal biopsies. However, if cyclosporin has to be continued because of the severity of the psoriasis and inability to control the disease with other drugs, then renal biopsy should probably be performed if the renal function tests imply a significant decrease in function, so that an accurate assessment of nephrotoxicity can be made.

Advantages   Cyclosporin is a highly effective treatment for psoriasis. It has less subjective side-effects than methotrexate and etretinate and is, therefore, preferred by the patients.

Disadvantages   The minor side-effects that patients may experience are nausea, paraesthesia and hypertrichosis. However, these are usually not severe and do not necessitate cessation of therapy. The two main problems associated with cyclosporin are hypertension and nephrotoxicity. There are two clinical patterns of hypertension associated with cyclosporin. In the first, the hypertension develops within the first 3 months of starting treatment and the incidence is approximately 15%. In the second pattern, hypertension develops after long-term treatment, i.e. after 2 years or more. The incidence of hypertension developing late in treatment is related to duration of therapy. Thus after 2 years, the incidence is approximately 30% and at 5 years 40%. Fortunately, the hypertension associated with cyclosporin is not severe, and can be controlled with hypotensive agents. The calcium channel blocker, nifedipine, is the most suitable drug with which to initiate hypotensive treatment. The hypertension due to cyclosporin is reversible when the drug is discontinued.

The second problem associated with cyclosporin is nephrotoxicity. Cyclosporin causes constriction of the renal arteriole and this there may be an immediate but small decrease in renal function. If cyclosporin is continued for long periods, there may be structural changes in the kidney, consisting of tubular atrophy, increased interstitial fibrosis, hyaline deposits in the renal arterioles and an increase in glomerular obsolescence. Severe renal damage should be preventable by close monitoring of patients and cessation of therapy if necessary.

All patients who are immunosuppressed run a risk of increased malignancy and, therefore, this is a potential hazard with cyclosporin treatment. To date, there has been no significant increase in malignancy associated with cyclosporin for psoriasis, but the duration of treatment is relatively short.

Efficacy   Cyclosporin is a very effective drug for clearing psoriasis.

Indications   Cyclosporin should be reserved for severe chronic plaque disease (unresponsive to topical measures and ultraviolet light treatments), erythrodermic, localized pustular psoriasis and generalized pustular psoriasis.

Contraindications Cyclosporin is contraindicated in cases of impaired renal function, malignancy and chronic infections.

Other systemic drugs

Both hydroxyurea and azathioprine have been used in the past. However, azathioprine is not very effective, and, although hydroxyurea has a better therapeutic effect, it is not as good as methotrexate or cyclosporin. In addition, hydroxyurea frequently causes bone marrow suppression.

Systemic steroids should not, as a general rule, be used for psoriasis. There is always a risk of 'rebound' when the steroids are reduced. Systemic steroids have been used in high dosage (e.g. 100 mg prednisolone daily) for erythrodermic psoriasis, but cyclosporin or methotrexate are now usually preferred.

Combined treatments

Therapeutic agents for psoriasis are often combined, first, because they may have a synergistic effect, and second, to decrease the side-effects of one, or both, of the treatments.

Coal tar and ultraviolet light

This combination has been used for many years and enhances the speed of clearance compared to the individual modalities.

Etretinate and photochemotherapy

Etretinate has been shown to lower the amount of UVA in PUVA treatment necessary to clear psoriasis. However, even if etretinate is only taken for a few weeks, female patients of childbearing age have to avoid pregnancy for 2 years. Another drawback is that patients usually develop cheilitis and dryness of the skin.

Systemic drugs and topical treatment

Not infrequently, a few resistant plaques of psoriasis may remain when patients are treated with cyclosporin, methotrexate or etretinate. If these patches are a nuisance to the patient, it may be possible to clear them with the addition of topical steroids or calcipotriol rather than to increase the dose of the systemic drug.

A combination of the current systemic drugs is not advisable because of the increased risk of side-effects.

Future treatments

Over the last decade there have been significant discoveries in the pathogenesis of psoriasis. There is now conclusive evidence that T lymphocytes play a central role in the development of the disease. The introduction of the use of cyclosporin and the new immunosuppressive drug FK-506 for the treatment of psoriasis was based on the role of the T lymphocyte in the disease process. There are two other important observations relating to the pathogenesis of psoriasis which may open up new treatments. First, psoriasis is probably an antigen-driven disease and, therefore, antigen-presenting cells play an important role; second, the 'end-organ' in psoriasis appears to be the keratinocyte. The lymphocytes produce cytokines which initiate the keratinocyte proliferation.

Thus future treatments may be directed against the antigen-presenting cell, the lymphocyte, or the keratinocyte.

The HLA class II antigen on the surface of antigen-presenting cells plays an important role in antigen presentation. Techniques to block antigen presentation, if selective, would inhibit this part of the pathogenic pathway.

It is likely that a specific clone of T cell is involved in psoriasis. If this clone is identified, it is possible that a specific monoclonal antibody would selectively block the action of this T cell clone. Another approach which may prove fruitful is to block the receptor on the T cells with peptides, which themselves would not stimulate the cells, but would not allow stimulation by the peptides of the specific antigen which they recognize. The T cell receptor is specific for a peptide, and this specificity depends on its structure. If the T cell receptor is cloned, then it may be possible to develop monoclonal antibodies to block the receptor.

Finally, anti-cytokines or monoclonal antibodies which block receptors, to cytokines on keratinocytes would interfere with the keratinocyte proliferation. Alternatively, a cytokine which inhibits keratinocyte proliferation might prove to be helpful in reversing the psoriatic process.

All these treatments are speculative, but are theoretically feasible. The selectivity of the treatment is of the utmost importance so that cells concerned with normal immunological function are not affected. Future treatments will undoubtedly depend on a greater understanding of the disease at a molecular level.

Section 2 Psoriasis Illustrated

List of Illustrations

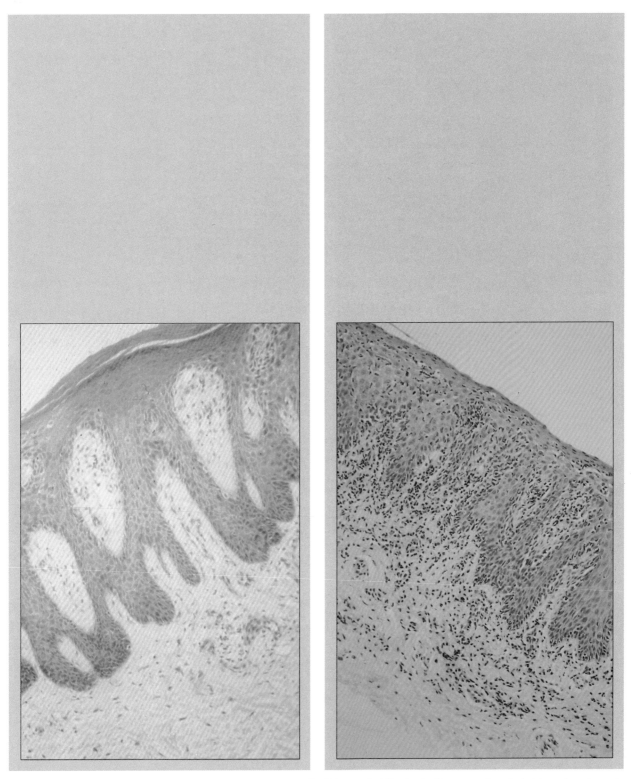

Figure 1 Histological features of psoriasis. Hyperplasia of the epidermis. Poorly-formed granular layer, hyperkeratosis and parakeratosis of the stratum corneum. Collection of neutrophils in the epidermis

Figure 2 Histological features of psoriasis. Heavy lymphocytic infiltrate of the dermis

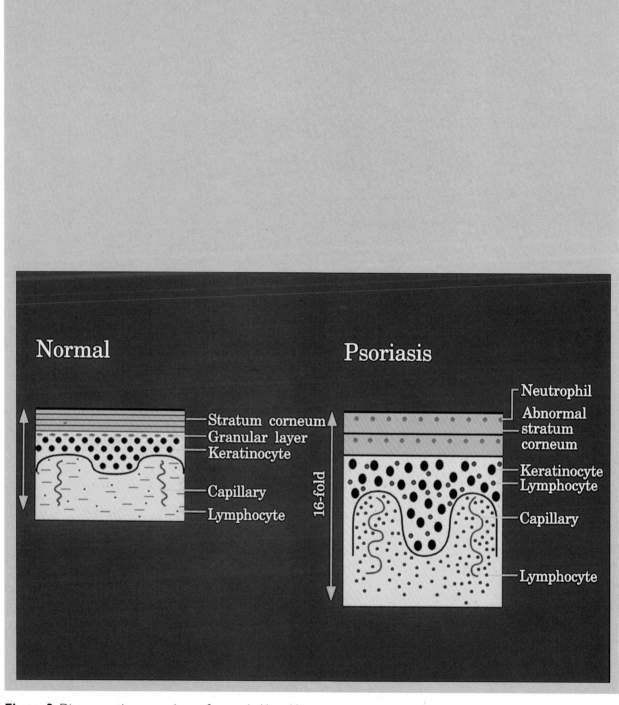

Figure 3 Diagrammatic comparison of normal skin with established psoriasis. There is a 16-fold increase in the thickness of the skin in psoriasis

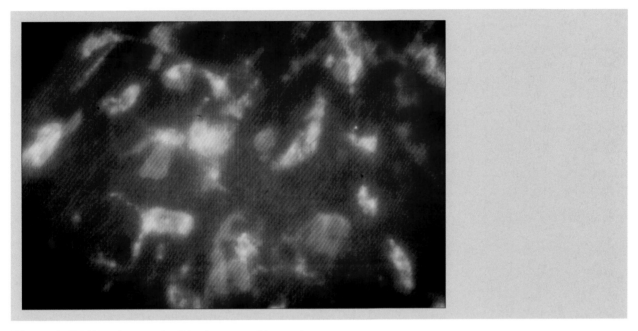

Figure 4 CD4 lymphocytes (red) in close apposition to the dendritic processes (green) of the antigen-presenting cells (Langerhans cells) in the initiation of guttate psoriasis

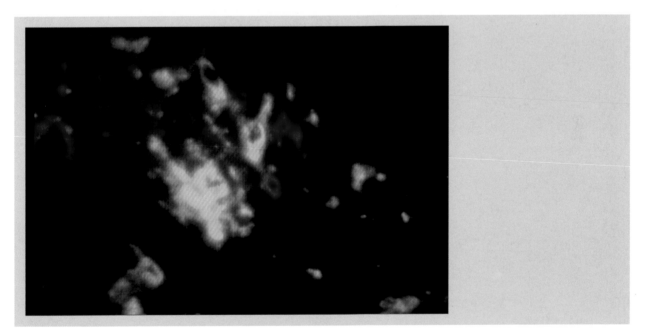

Figure 5 CD8 lymphocytes (red) in close apposition to the dendritic processes (green) of antigen-presenting cells in the resolution of guttate psoriasis

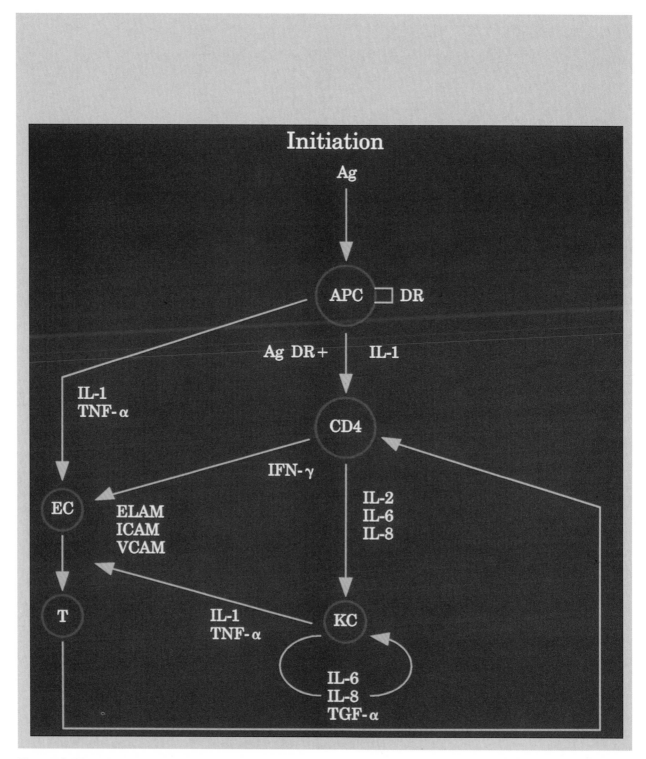

Figure 6 Diagrammatic representation of cells and cytokines involved in the initiation of psoriasis. EC = endothelial cell; APC = antigen-presenting cell; T = T lymphocyte; KC = keratinocyte

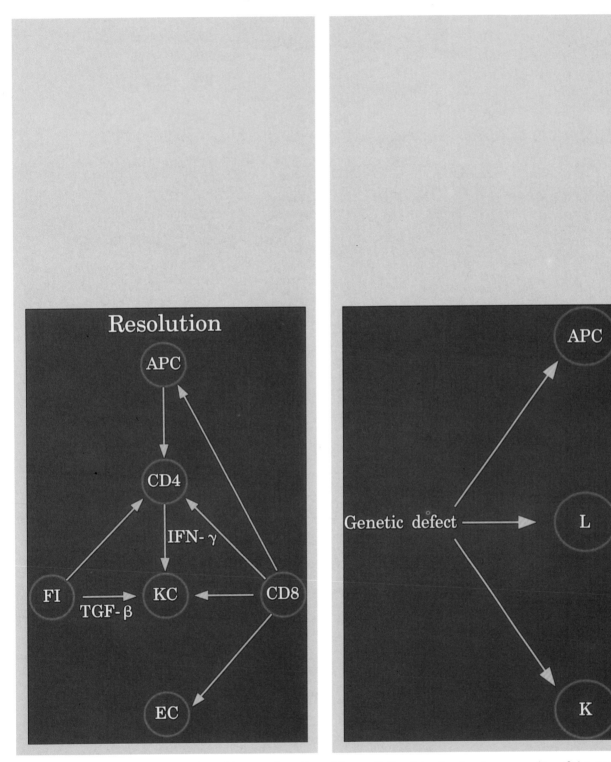

Figure 7 Possible sites of action of cytokines produced by CD8 (suppressor) lymphocytes in the resolution of psoriasis. EC = endothelial cell; KC = keratinocyte; APC = antigen-presenting cell; FI = fibroblast

Figure 8 Possible sites for the expression of the genetic defect in psoriasis. APC = antigen-presenting cell; L = lymphocyte; K = keratinocyte

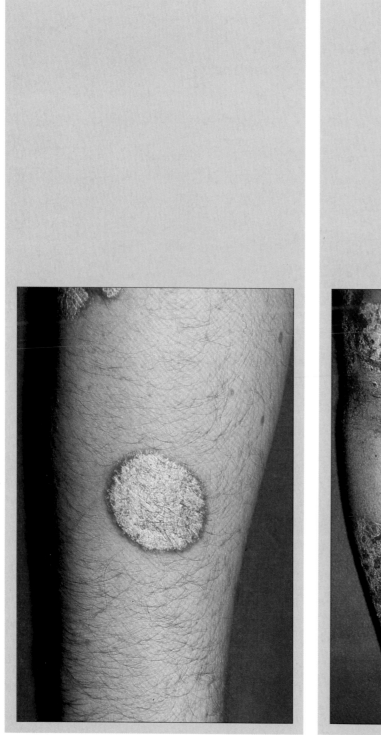

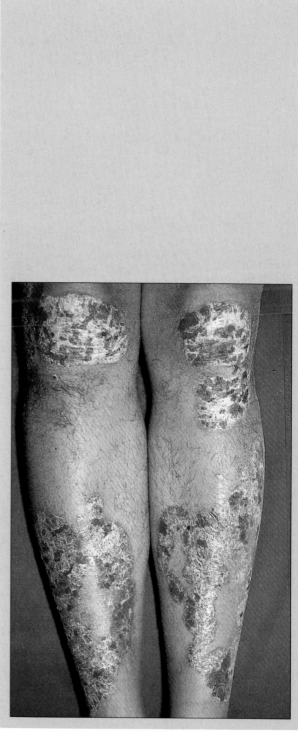

Figure 9 Sharply demarcated plaque with white scale

Figure 10 Symmetrical red plaques of psoriasis with minimal scaling

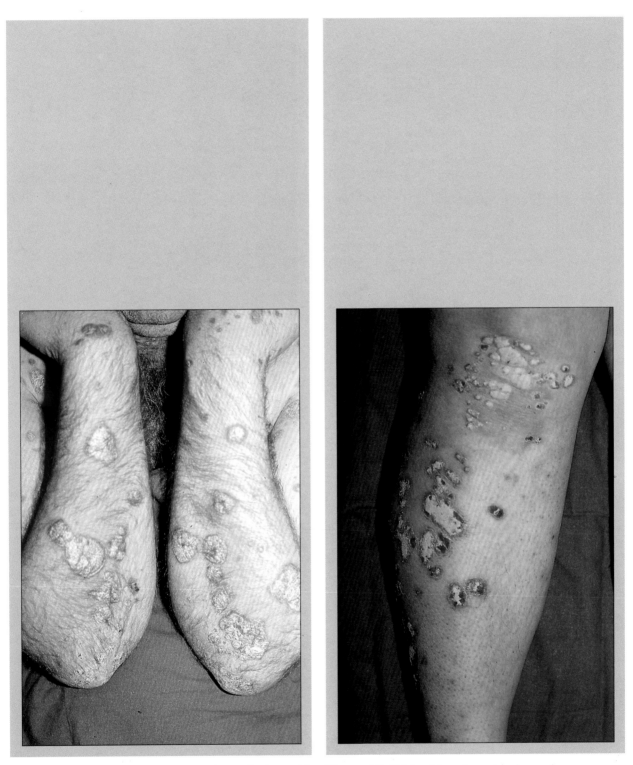

Figure 11 Thick plaques some with white, and others with grey scale

Figure 12 Thick, white adherent scale on plaques

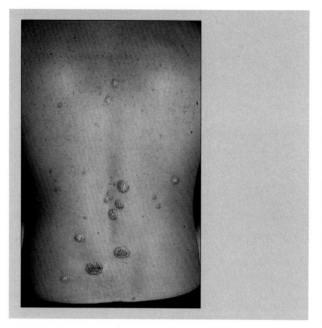

Figure 13 Dark grey scale in untreated, chronic, plaque psoriasis

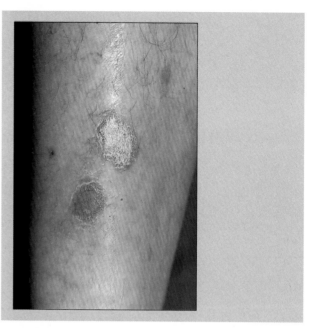

Figure 14 Excoriation of a plaque converting a red, non-scaly surface into a white, scaly one

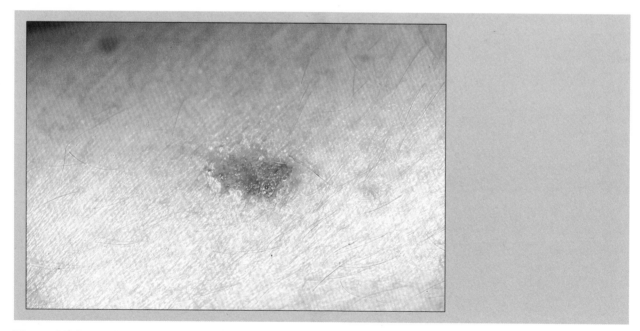

Figure 15 Patch of psoriasis with the scale removed showing a glistening surface

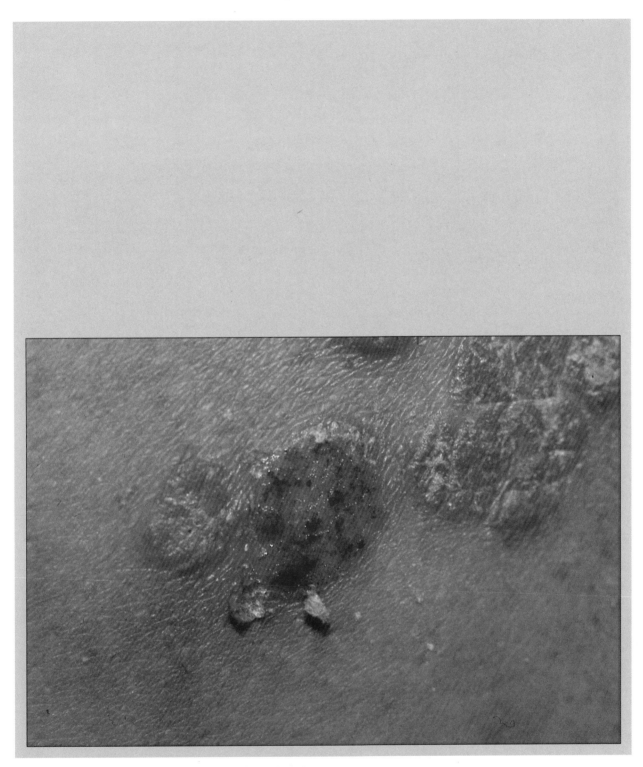

Figure 16 Capillary bleeding after removal of scale in active
psoriasis

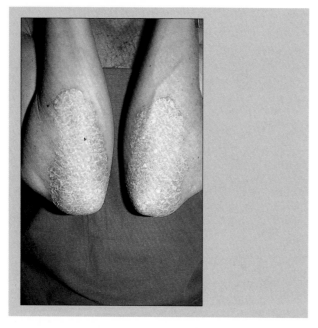

Figure 17 Symmetrical plaques on one of the common sites, the elbows

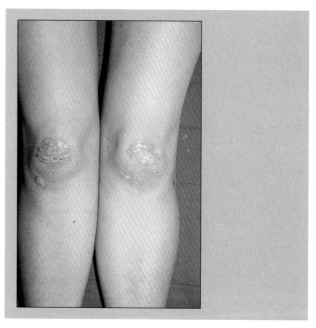

Figure 18 Symmetrical plaques on a common site, the knees

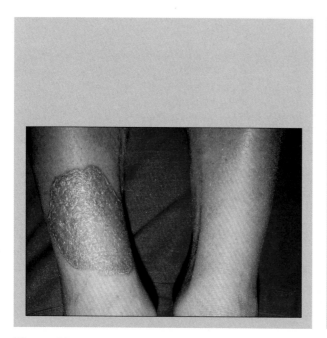

Figure 19 Unilateral psoriasis. An unusual presentation

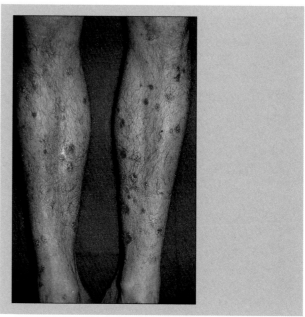

Figure 20 Numerous small plaques

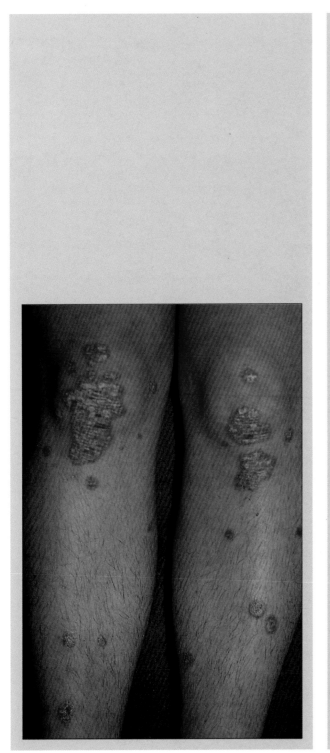

Figure 21 Small and moderate-sized plaques

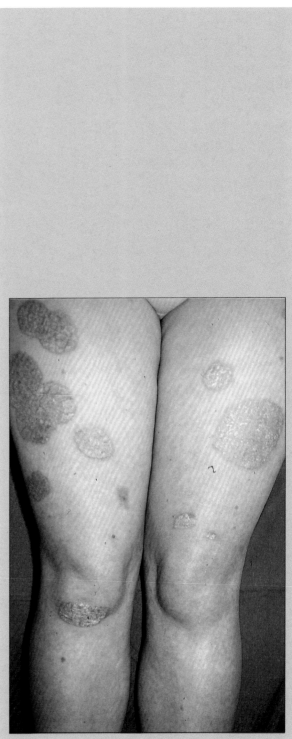

Figure 22 Plaques of various sizes with minimal scale on the thighs

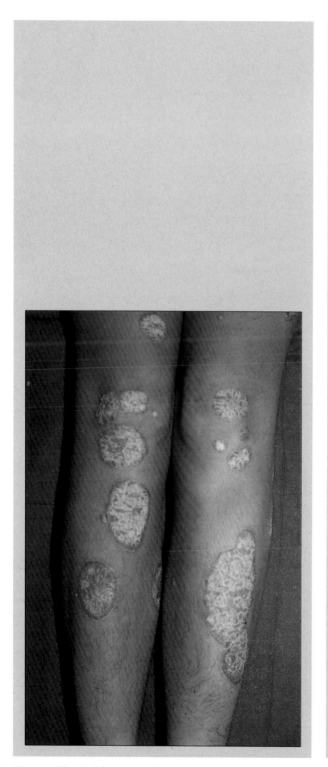

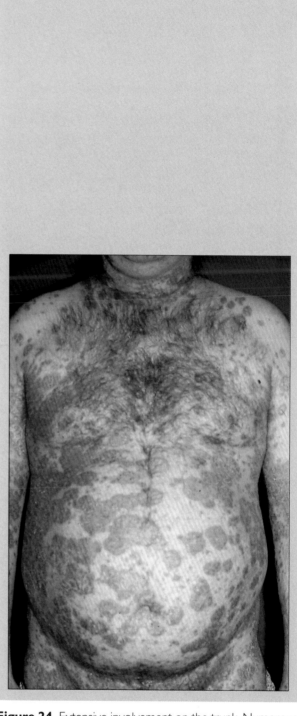

Figure 23 Various-sized plaques with white scale on the legs

Figure 24 Extensive involvement on the trunk. Numerous large plaques

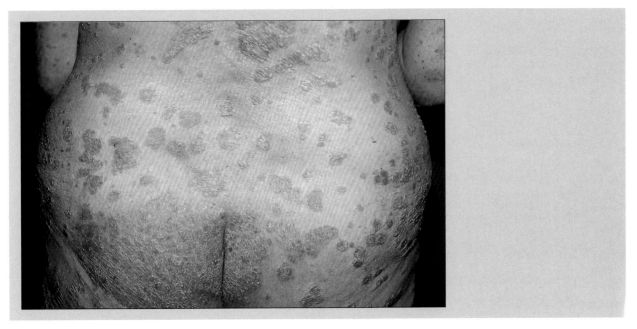

Figure 25 Large and small plaques on the lower back

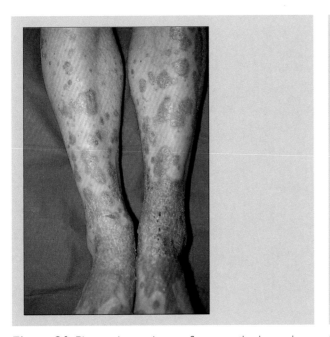

Figure 26 Plaques becoming confluent on the lower legs

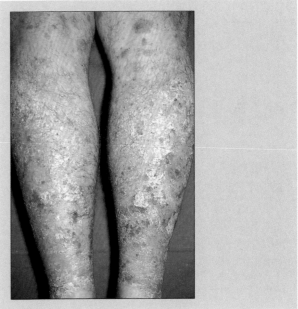

Figure 27 Confluent psoriasis on the back of the legs

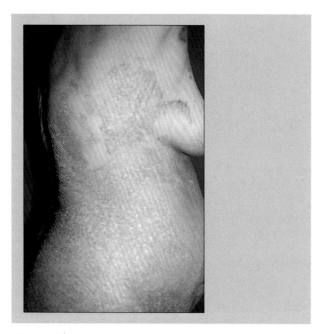

Figure 28 Extensive confluent psoriasis on the trunk

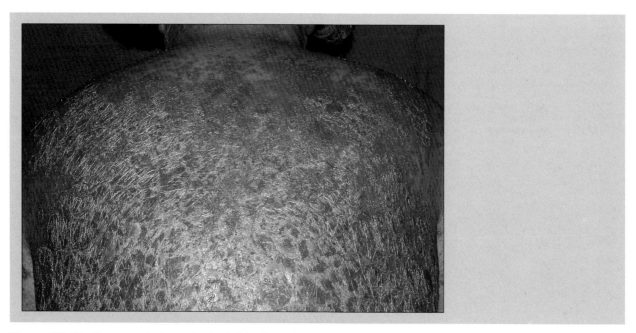

Figure 29 Confluent psoriasis on the back. Nearly all the skin is involved

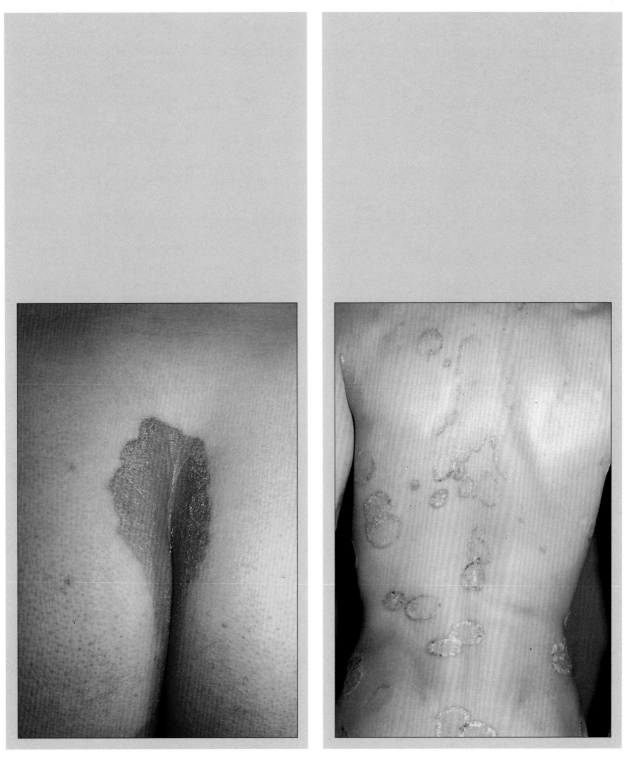

Figure 30 Psoriasis over the sacral area, another common site for psoriasis

Figure 31 Resolving psoriasis, presenting as annular lesions

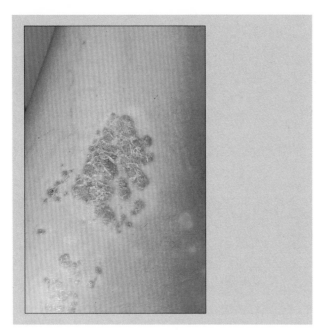

Figure 32 Loss of pigment where psoriasis has cleared

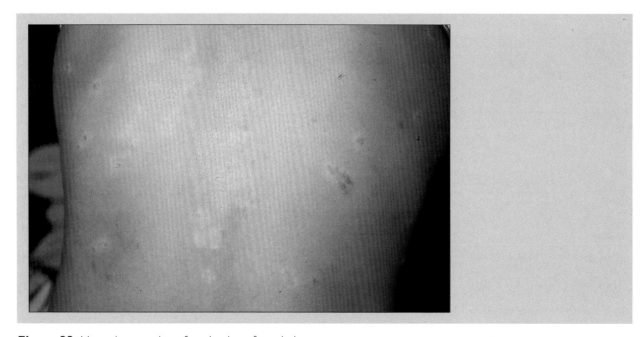

Figure 33 Hypopigmentation after clearing of psoriasis

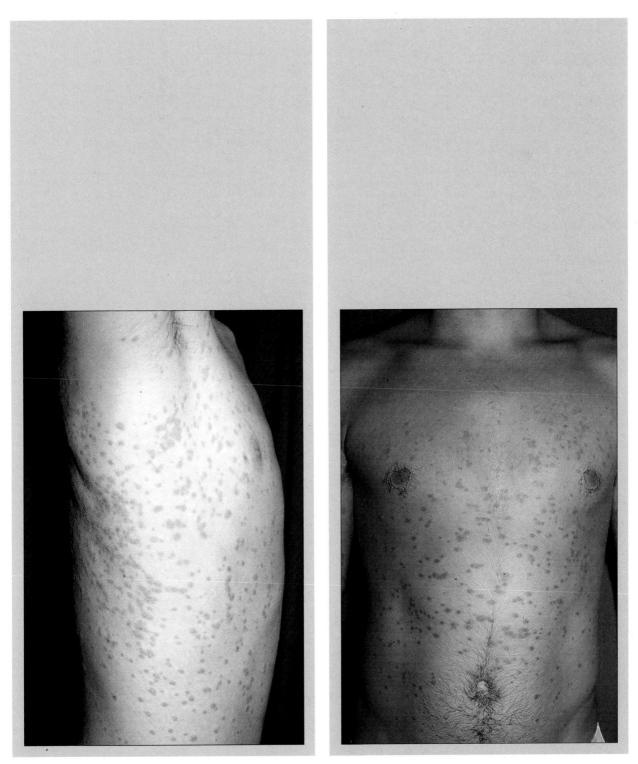

Figure 34 Guttate psoriasis. A mild form with a few lesions on the trunk

Figure 35 Guttate psoriasis on the chest and upper abdomen

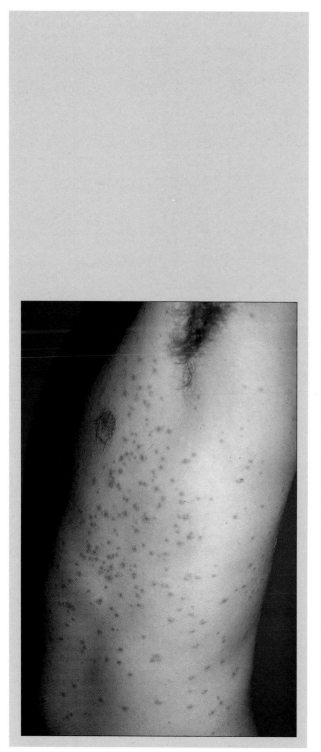

Figure 36 Guttate psoriasis on the side of the trunk

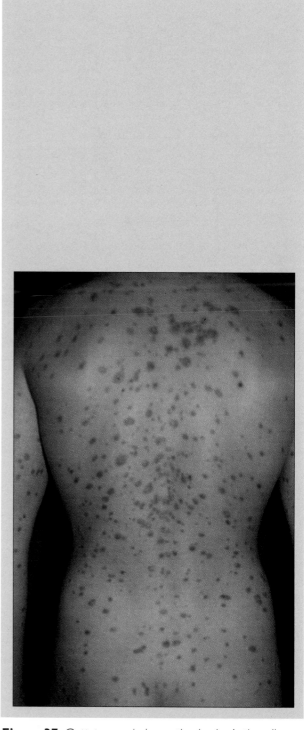

Figure 37 Guttate psoriasis on the back. Active disease with lesions showing a tendency to enlarge

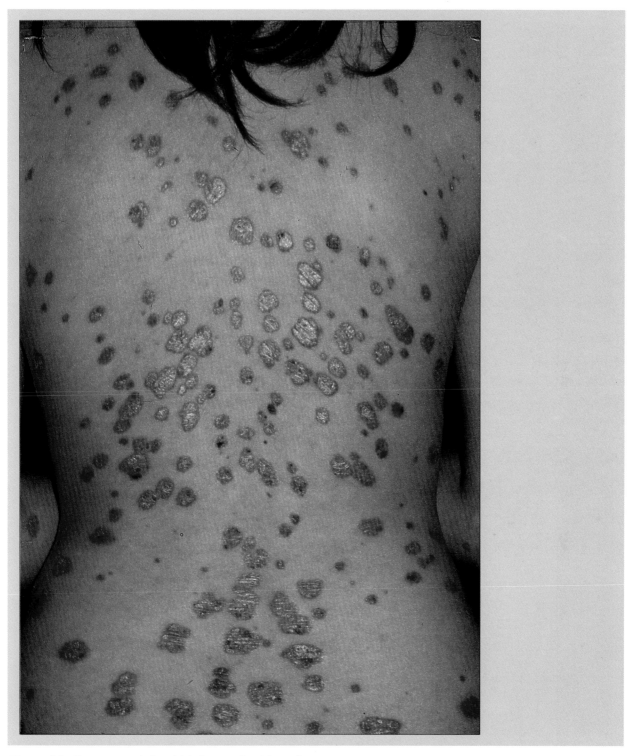

Figure 38 Guttate psoriasis which has evolved into the plaque form

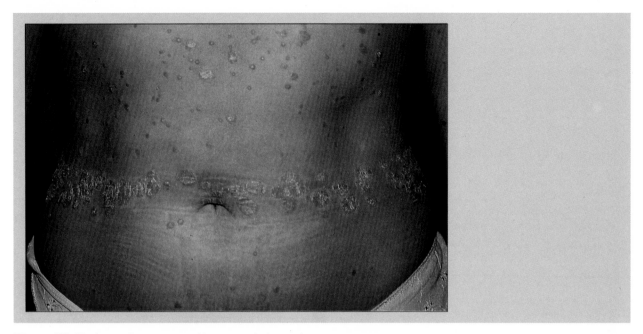

Figure 39 Koebner phenomenon. Linear psoriasis on the waist from tight clothing

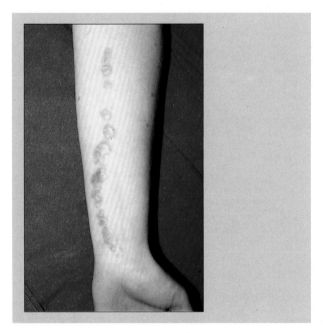

Figure 40 Koebner positive. Linear psoriasis from a scratch

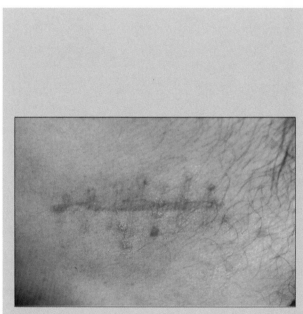

Figure 41 Koebner phenomenon. Psoriasis at an operation site, particularly at the sites of the sutures

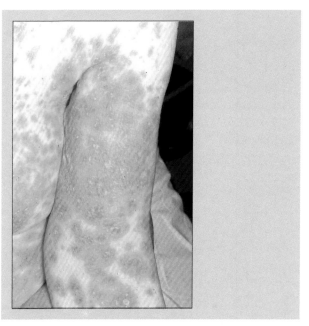

Figure 43 Generalized pustular psoriasis. Numerous, small pustules on the arm

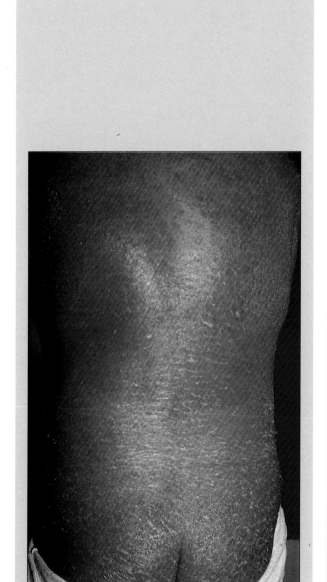

Figure 42 Erythrodermic psoriasis

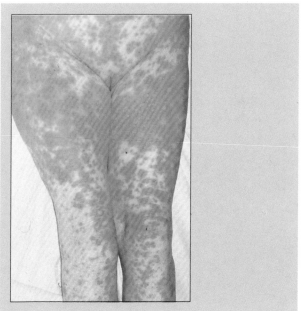

Figure 44 Generalized pustular psoriasis. Pustules on the thighs

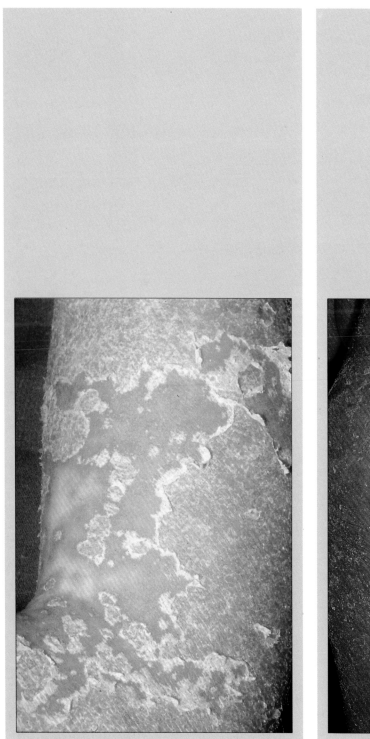

Figure 45 Resolving, pustular psoriasis

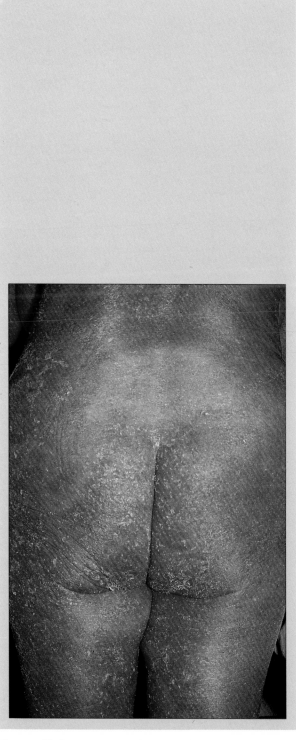

Figure 46 Erythroderma following generalized pustular psoriasis

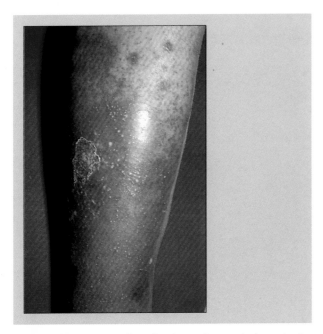

Figure 47 An area of localized pustular psoriasis on the leg

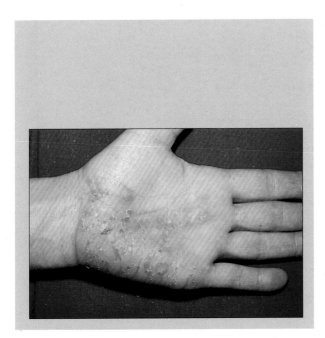

Figure 48 Localized pustular psoriasis on the palm, erythema and scaling

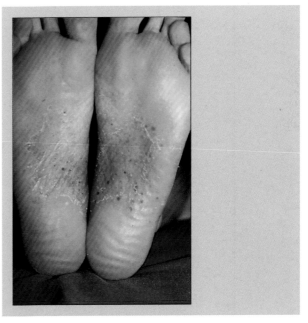

Figure 49 Symmetrical localized pustular psoriasis on the soles

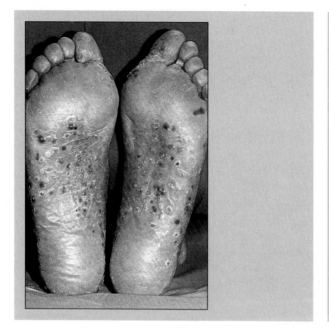

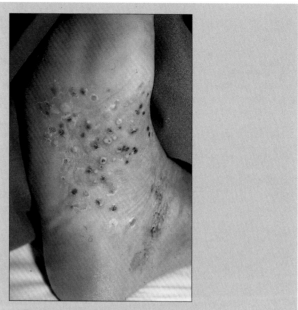

Figure 50 Pustules and 'brown papules', characteristic of localized pustular psoriasis on the soles

Figure 51 Severe pustulation in localized pustular psoriasis

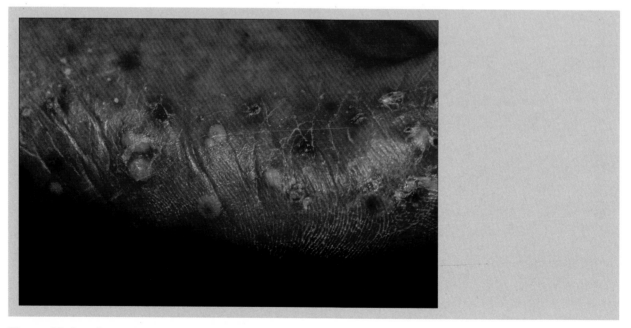

Figure 52 Pustular psoriasis on the side of the foot

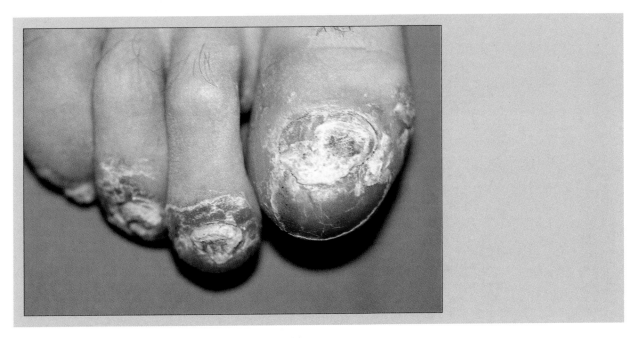

Figure 53 Acral psoriasis. Severe nail dystrophy and involvement of the nail folds

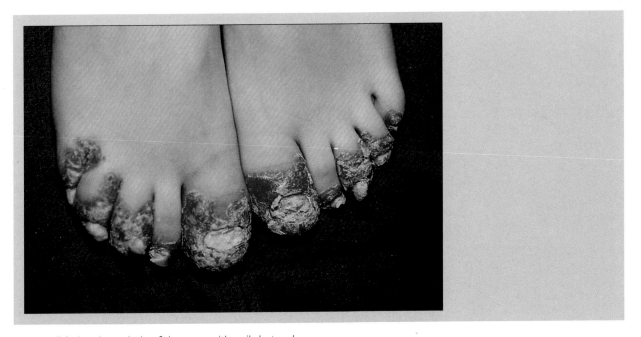

Figure 54 Acral psoriasis of the toes with nail dystrophy

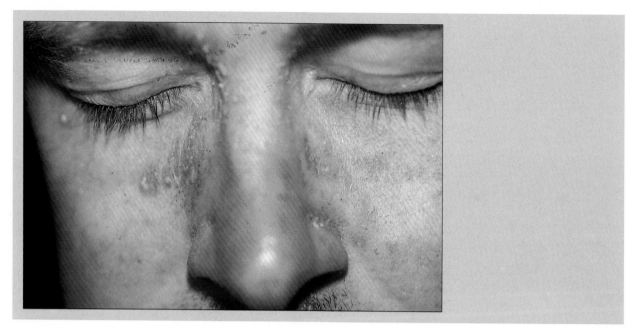

Figure 55 Psoriasis on the face at the typical sites of seborrhoeic eczema (seborrhoeic psoriasis)

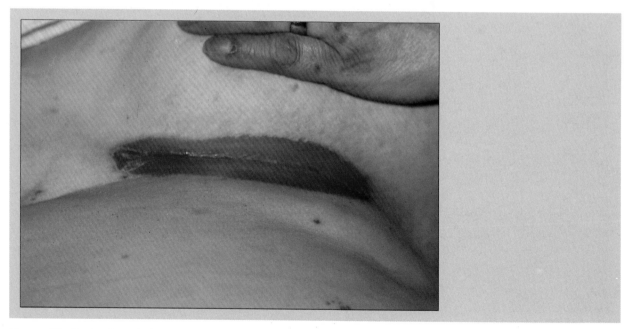

Figure 56 Patch of psoriasis under the breast

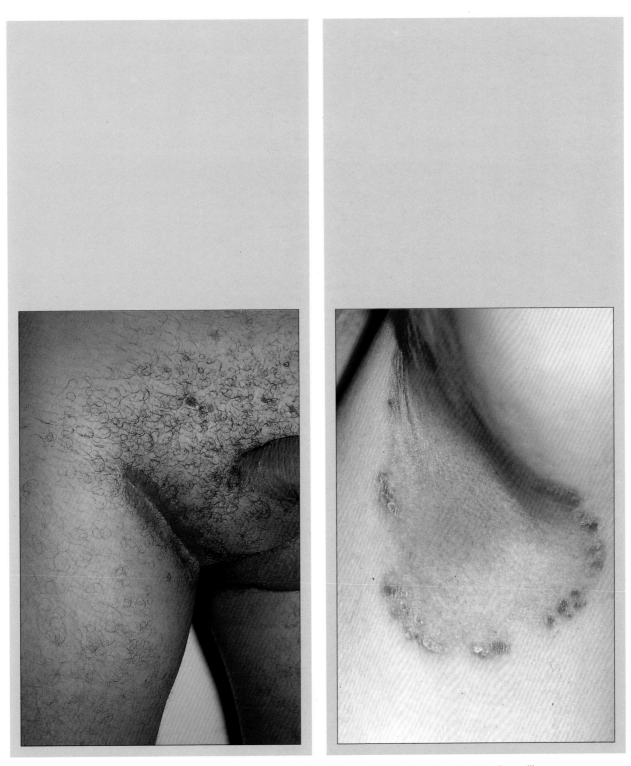

Figure 57 Psoriasis localized to the intertrigenous area of the groin

Figure 58 Psoriasis localized to the axilla

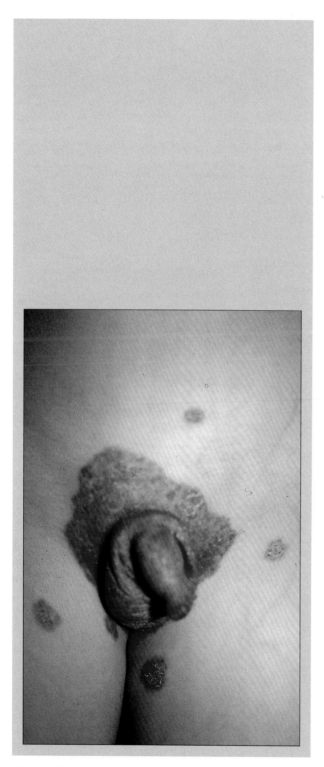

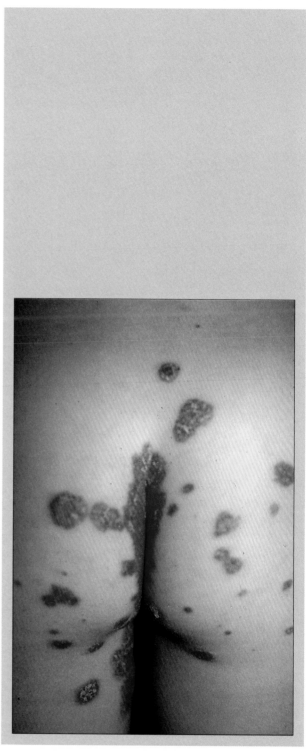

Figure 59 Psoriasis of the genitalia and pubic area, common sites in children

Figure 60 Psoriasis of the natal cleft (a common site in children), with surrounding plaques

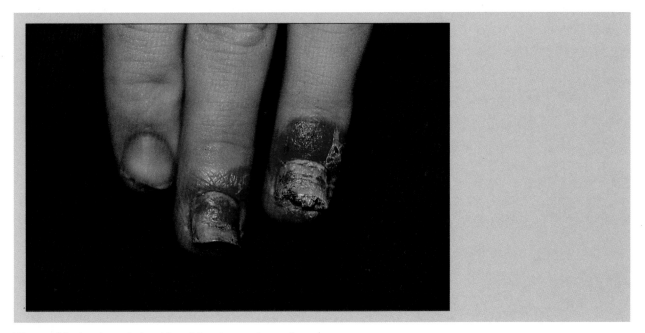

Figure 61 Acral psoriasis with nail involvement, a not un-common presentation in childhood

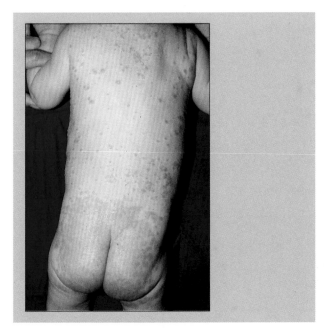

Figure 62 Confluent involvement in napkin area, and papules and plaques on the trunk in napkin 'psoriasis'

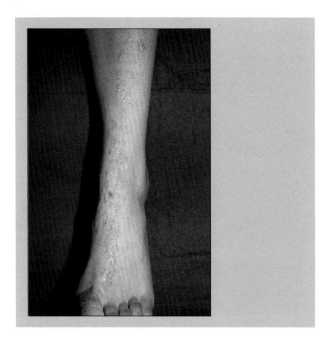

Figure 63 Linear psoriasis

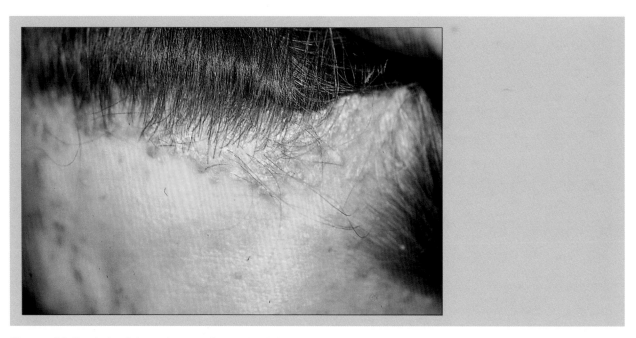

Figure 64 Psoriasis of the scalp extending to the hairline

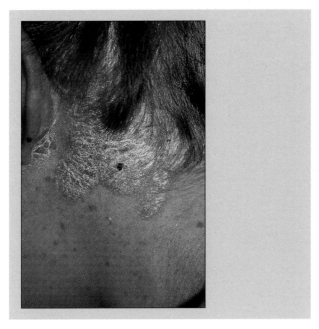

Figure 65 Extension of psoriasis just beyond the hairline in active disease

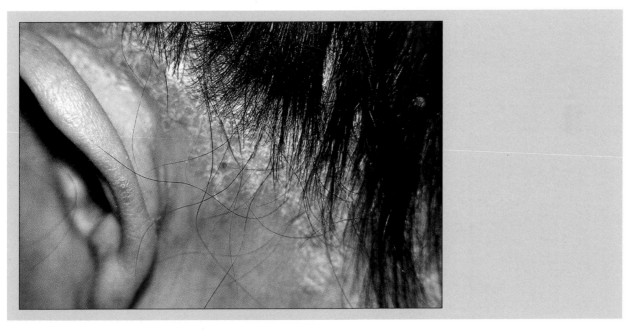

Figure 66 A common site of scalp psoriasis, behind the ear

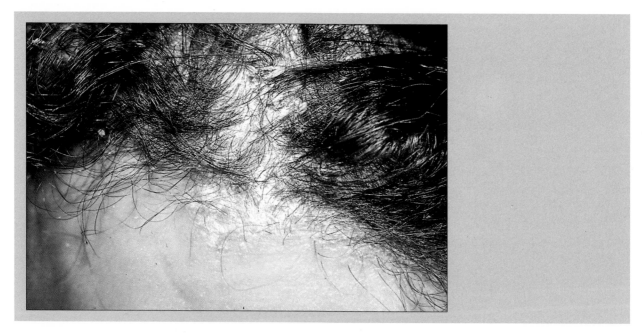

Figure 67 Thick scales of scalp psoriasis

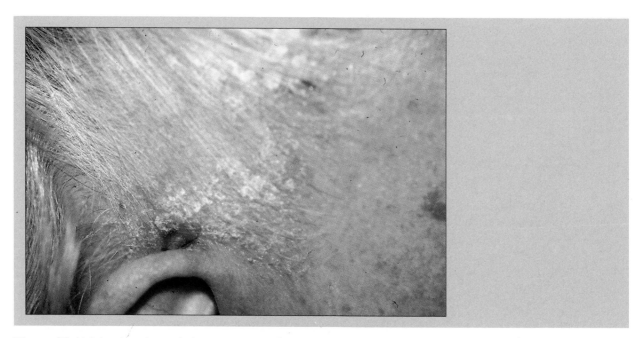

Figure 68 Hair loss in scalp psoriasis, an uncommon feature

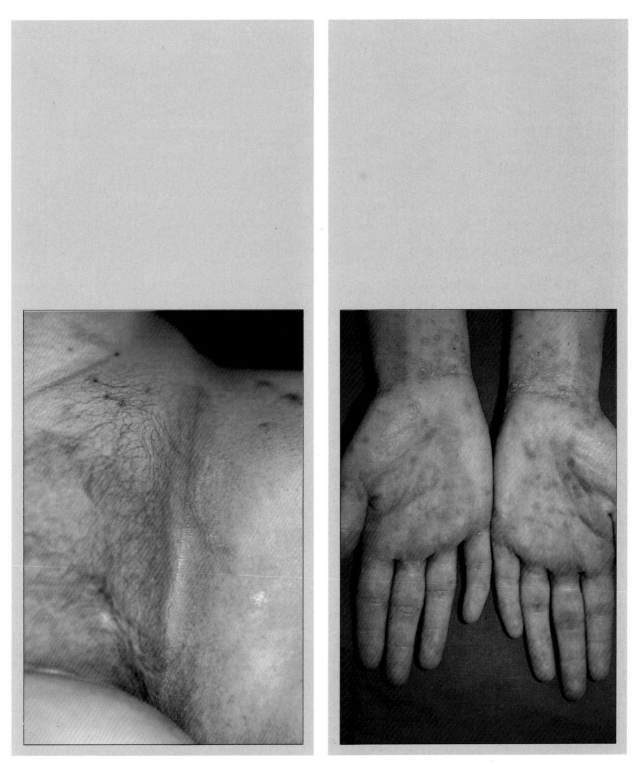

Figure 69 Psoriasis localized to the pubic area

Figure 70 Guttate psoriasis on the palms

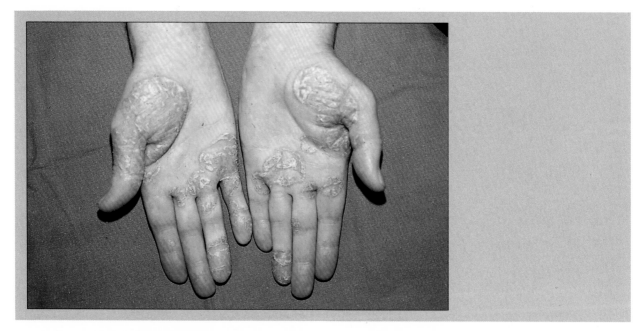

Figure 71 Localized symmetrical lesions of psoriasis on the palms. The scaling is different to plaque psoriasis elsewhere on the trunk and limbs

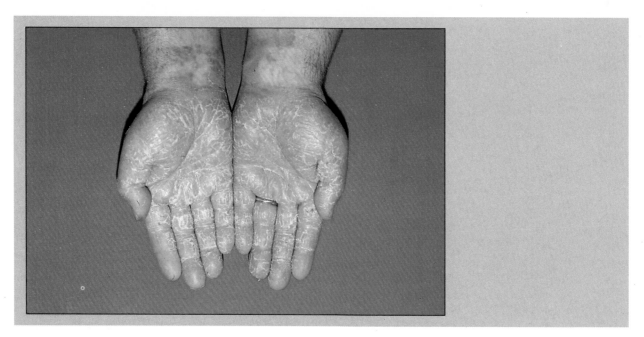

Figure 72 Confluent psoriasis on the palms

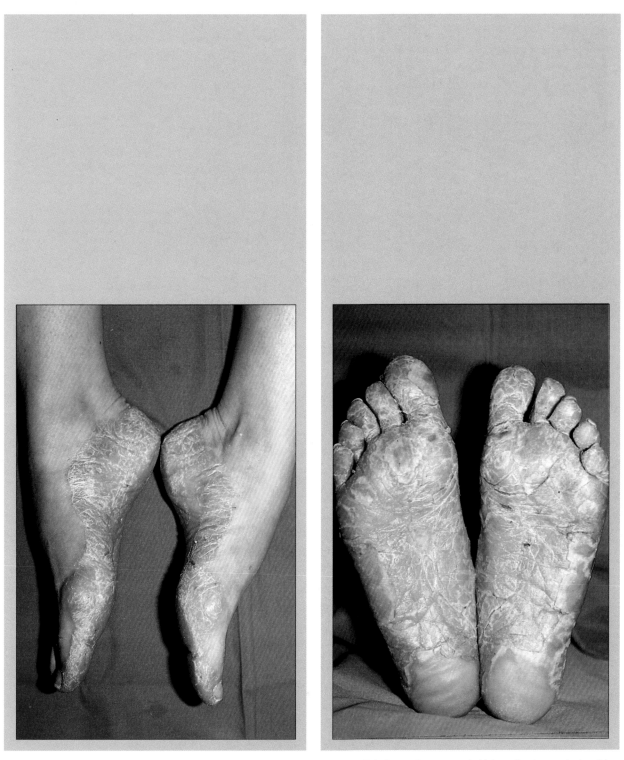

Figure 73 Sharp line of demarcation between psoriasis on the sole and the surrounding skin

Figure 74 Deep fissures and thick scales in psoriasis of the soles

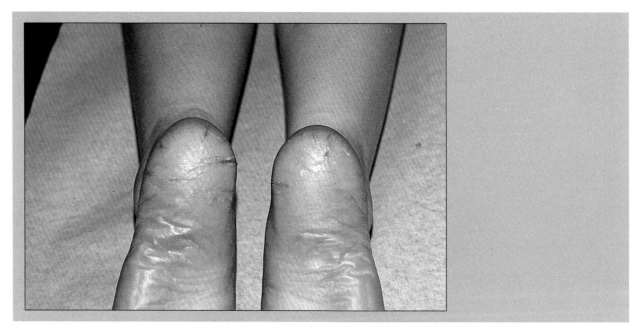

Figure 75 Fissuring in psoriasis of the soles

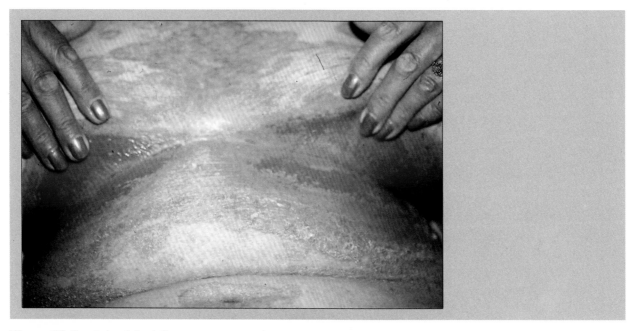

Figure 76 Psoriasis of the infra-mammary areas in extensive plaque disease

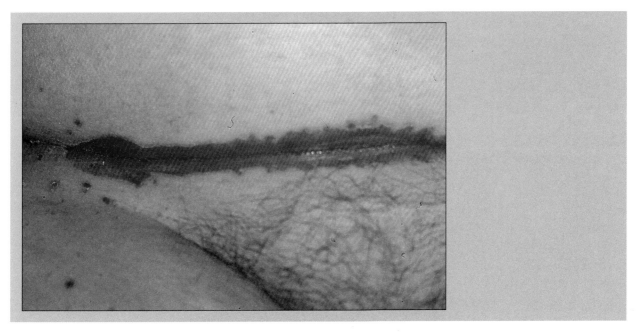

Figure 77 Psoriasis confined to the intertrigenous area of an abdominal fold. Fissuring is present

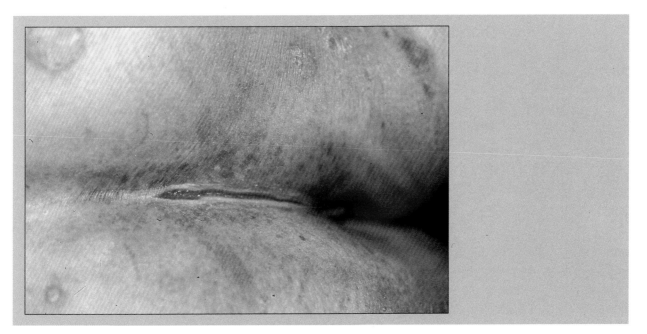

Figure 78 Deep fissure of the natal cleft

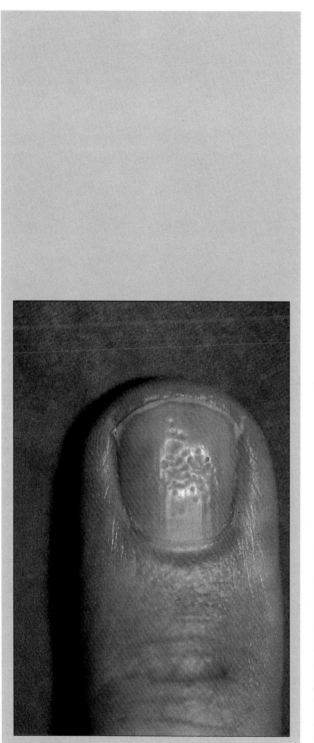

Figure 79 Pits in the nail

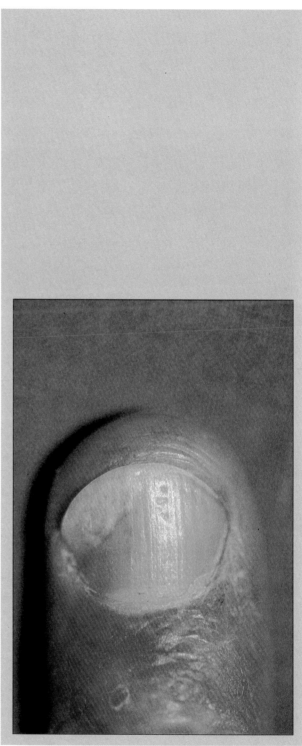

Figure 80 Pitting and onycholysis of the nail plate

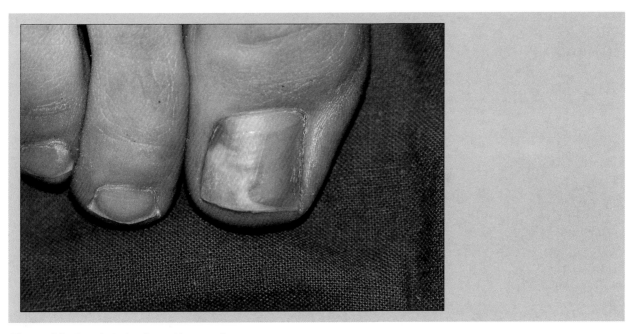

Figure 81 Onycholysis of one big toenail

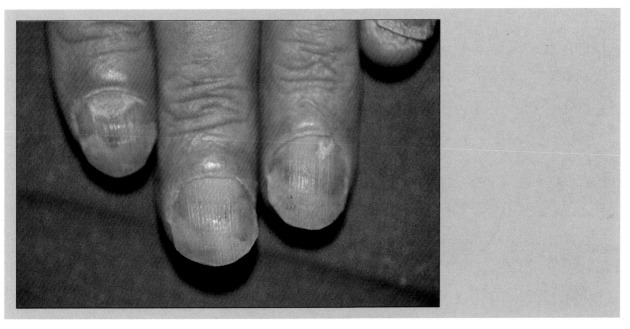

Figure 82 Severe onycholysis

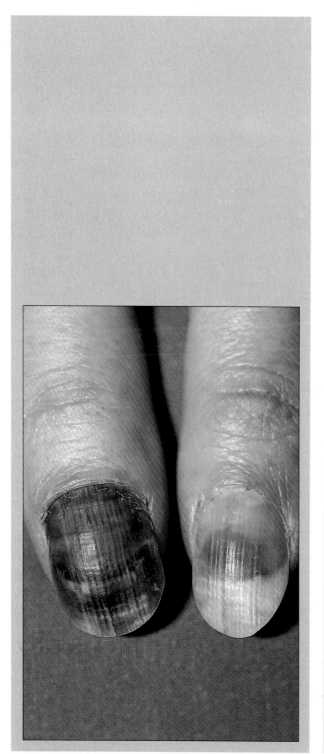

Figure 83 Greenish discoloration due to chromogenic bacteria under the nail in onycholysis

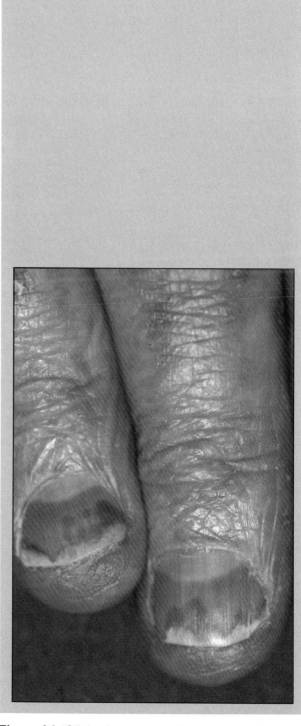

Figure 84 'Oil drop' appearance due to psoriasis of the nail bed

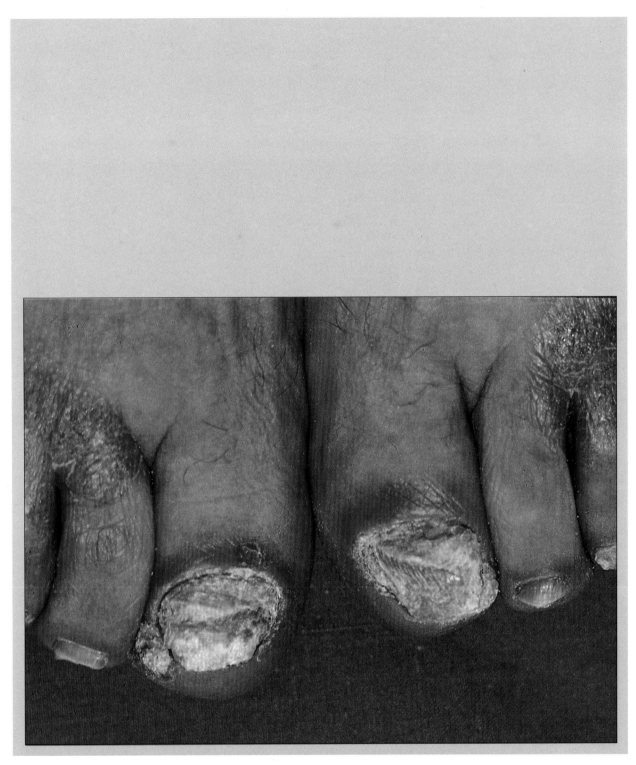

Figure 85 Subungual hyperkeratosis and dystrophy of the nail plate

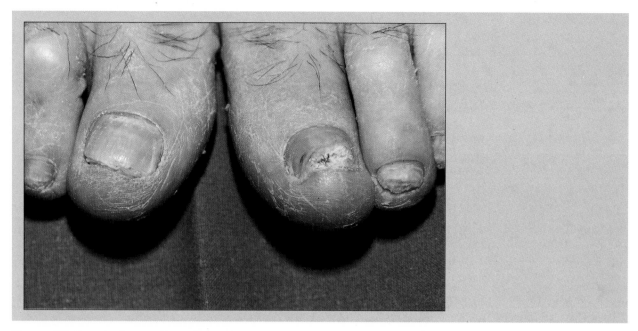

Figure 86 Severe subungual hyperkeratosis

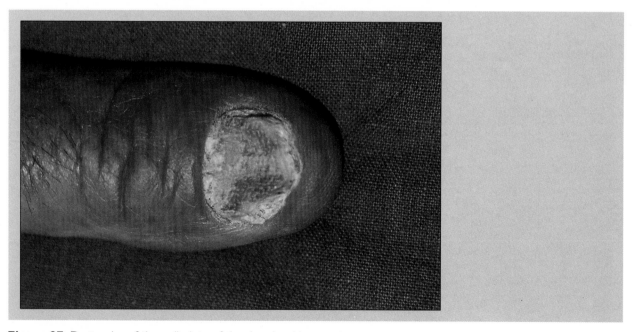

Figure 87 Dystrophy of the nail plate of the thumb with some subungual hyperkeratosis

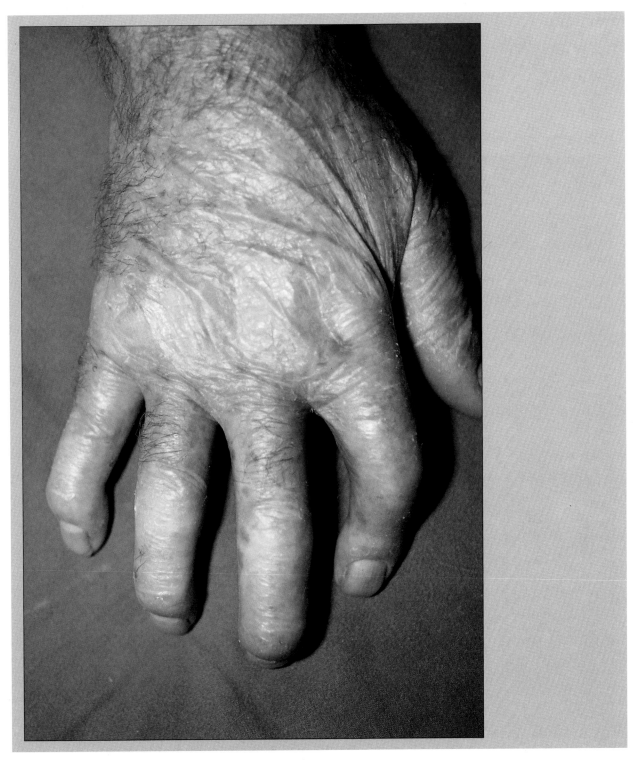

Figure 88 Psoriatic arthritis of the hand, involving both the proximal and distal interphalangeal joints. The latter is characteristic of psoriatic arthropathy

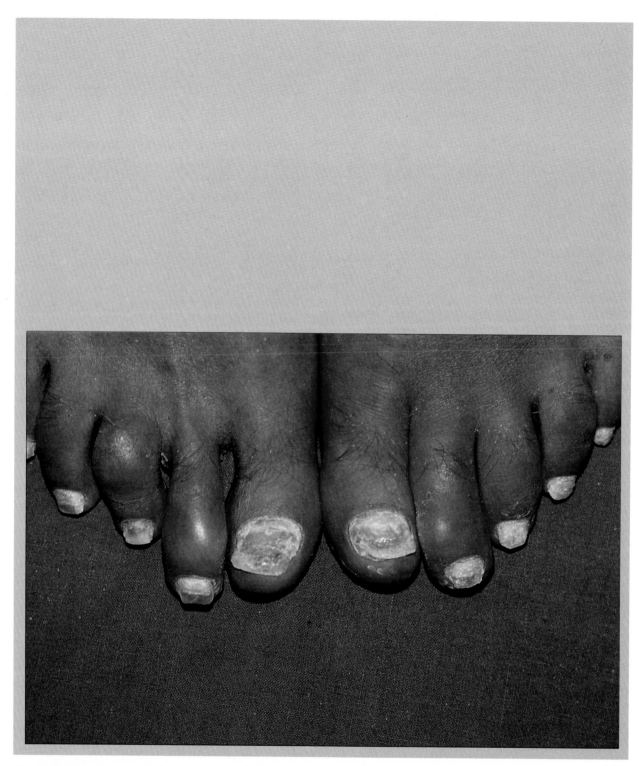

Figure 89 Involvement of the proximal and distal inter-phalangeal joints of the toes

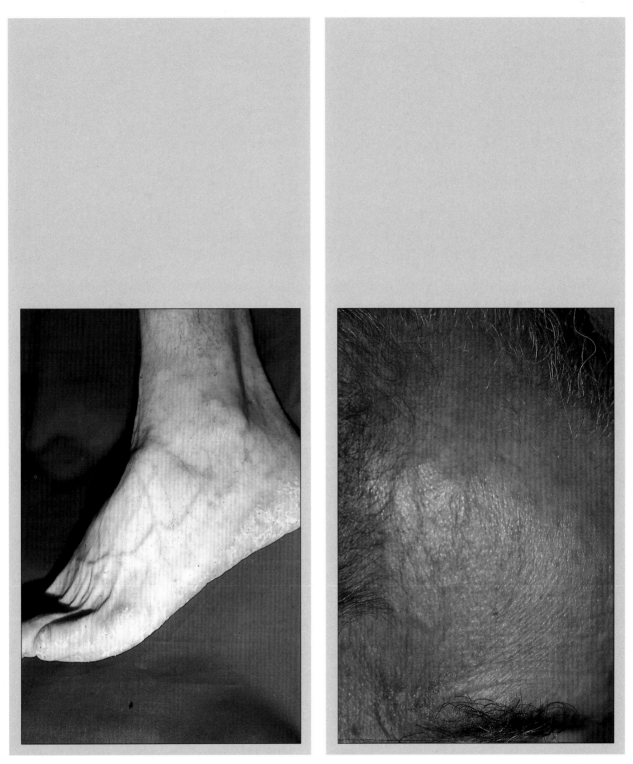

Figure 90 Thinning of the skin due to long-term use of potent, topical corticosteroids

Figure 91 Telangiectasia of the upper forehead following long-term use of a potent, topical steroid scalp lotion

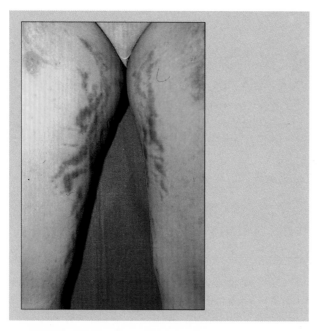

Figure 92 Striae on the thighs, following long-term use of a very potent topical steroid

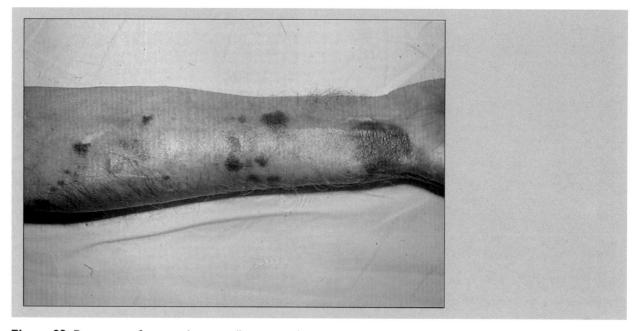

Figure 93 Purpura on forearm due to collagen atrophy after long-term potent steroids

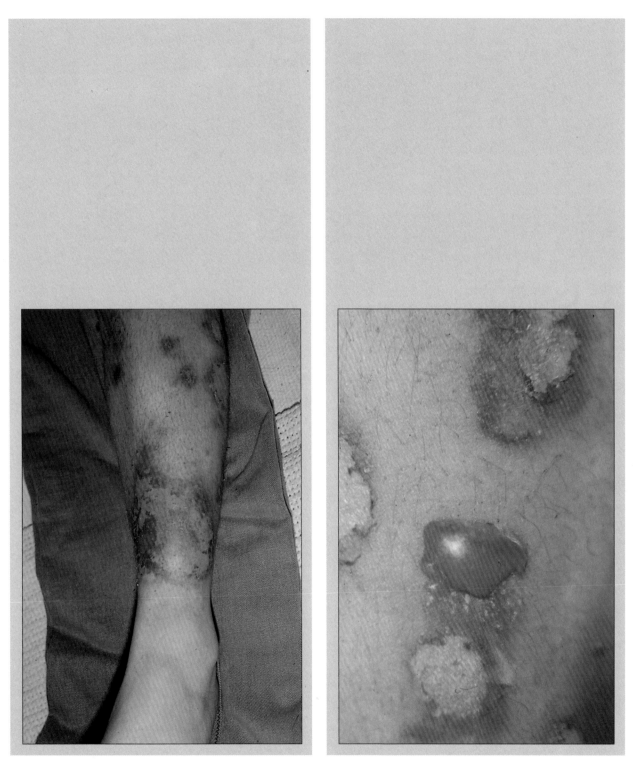

Figure 94 Dithranol staining: brownish discoloration of skin surrounding treated psoriatic plaque

Figure 95 Blisters, due to dithranol, on uninvolved skin surrounding a psoriatic plaque

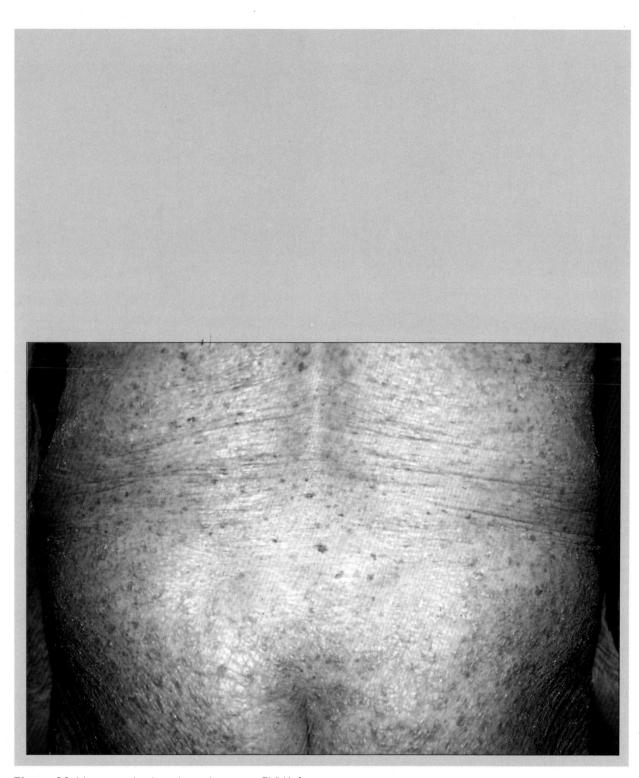

Figure 96 Numerous lentigos due to long-term PUVA for severe psoriasis

Section 3 Bibliography

Lomholt, G. (1963). *Psoriasis. Prevalence, Spontaneous Course and Genetics.* (Copenhagen: G. E. C. Gad)

Farber, E. M. and Nall, M. L. (1974). The natural history of psoriasis in 5000 patients. *Dermatologia,* **148**, 1–18

Williams, R. C., McKenzie, A. W., Roger, J. H. and Joysey, V. C. (1976). HL-A antigens in patients with guttate psoriasis. *Br. J. Dermatol.,* **95**, 163–7

Pedace, J., Muller, A. and Winkelmann, R. K. (1969). Biology of psoriasis: experimental study of Koebner phenomenon. *Acta Dermatovenerol.,* **49**, 390–400

Eyre, R. W. and Krueger, G. (1982). Response to injury of skin involved and uninvolved with psoriasis, and its relation to disease activity. *Br. J. Dermatol.,* **106**, 153–9

Baker, B. S., Swain, A. F., Fry, L. and Valdimarsson, H. (1984). Epidermal T lymphocytes and HLA-DR expression in psoriasis. *Br. J. Dermatol.,* **110**, 555–64

Baker, B. S., Powles, A. V., Lambert, S. *et al.* (1988). A prospective study of the Koebner reaction and T lymphocytes in uninvolved psoriatic skin. *Acta Dermatovenerol.,* **68**, 430–3

Norrlind, R. (1950). Psoriasis following infections with haemolytic streptococci. *Acta Dermatovenerol.,* **30**, 64–72

Norholm-Pederson, A. (1952). Infections and psoriasis. *Acta Dermatovenerol.,* **32**, 159–67

Swerlick, R. A., Cunningham, M. W. and Hall, N. K. (1986). Monoclonal antibodies cross-reactive with group A streptococci and normal and psoriatic human skin. *J. Invest. Dermatol.,* **87**, 367–71

Watson, W., Cann, H., Farber, E. *et al.* (1972). The genetics of psoriasis. *Arch. Dermatol.,* **105**, 197–207

Hellgren, L. (1967). *Psoriasis.* (Stockholm: Almqvist & Wiksell)

Bandrup, F., Hauge, M., Henningsen, K. and Eriksen, B. (1978). A study of psoriasis in unselected series of twins. *Arch. Dermatol.,* **114**, 874–8

Fry, L. and McMinn, R. M. H. (1968). The action of chemotherapeutic agents on psoriatic epidermis. *Br. J. Dermatol.,* **80**, 373–83

Bjerke, J. R., Krogh, H. K. and Matre, R. (1978). Characterisation of mononuclear cell infiltrates in psoriatic lesions. *J. Invest. Dermatol.,* **71**, 340–3

Baker, B. S., Swain, A. F., Valdimarsson, H. and Fry, L.

(1984). T cell subpopulations in the blood and skin of patients with psoriasis. *Br. J. Dermatol.*, **110**, 37–44

Valdimarsson, H., Baker, B. S., Jonsdittir, I. and Fry, L. (1986). Psoriasis: a disease of abnormal keratinocyte proliferation induced by T lymphocytes. *Immunol. Today*, **7**, 256–9

Goodwin, P. G., Hamilton, S. and Fry, L. (1973). A comparison of DNA synthesis and mitosis in uninvolved and involved psoriatic epidermis and normal epidermis. *Br. J. Dermatol.*, **89**, 613–18

Voorhees, J. J. and Duel, E. A. (1971). Psoriasis as a possible defect of the adenyl cyclase-cyclic AMP cascade. *Arch. Dermatol.*, **104**, 352–8

Krueger, G. D. (1981). Psoriasis: current concepts of its aetiology and pathogenesis. In Dobson, R. L. and Thiers, R. H. (eds.) *Year Book of Dermatology*. (Chicago: Year Book Medical Publishers Inc.)

Voorhees, J. J. (1983). Leukotrienes and other lipoxygenase products in the pathogenesis and therapy of psoriasis and other dermatoses. *Arch. Dermatol.*, **119**, 541–7

Tronnier, H. and Schule, N. (1973). Zur dermatologischen Therapie von Dermatosen mit Langwellingen UV nach Photosensibilisirung der Haut mit Methoxsalen, erste Ergebnisse bei Psoriasis Vulgaris. *Zeitschrift Haut Geshlecktskrankheiten*, **48**, 385–93

Parrish, J. A., Fitzpatrick, T. B., Tannenbaum, L. and Pathak, M. A. (1974). Photochemotherapy of psoriasis with oral methossalen and long wave ultraviolet light. *N. Engl. J. Med.*, **291**, 1207–11

Borel, J. F., Feurer, C., Gibner, H. U. and Stahelein, N. (1976). Biological effects of cyclosporin A: a new antilymphocytic agent. *Agents Actions*, **6**, 468–75

Griffiths, C. E. M., Powles, A. V., Leonard, J. N. *et al.*

(1986). Clearance of psoriasis with low dose cyclosporin. *Br. Med. J.*, **293**, 731–2

Powles, A. V., Baker, B. S., Valdimarsson, H., Hulme, B. and Fry, L. (1990). Four years of experience with cyclosporin A for psoriasis. *Br. J. Dermatol.*, **36**, 13–19

Fry, L. (1988). Psoriasis. *Br. J. Dermatol.*, **119**, 445–61

Baker, B. S., Brent, L., Valdimarsson, H., Powles, A. V., Al-Imara, L., Walker, M. and Fry, L. (1992). Is epidermal cell proliferation in psoriatic skin grafts on nude mice driven by T-cell derived cytokines? *Br. J. Dermatol.*, **126**, 105–10

Baker, B. S. and Fry, L. (1992). The immunology of psoriasis. *Br. J. Dermatol.*, **126**, 1–9

Mier, P. D. and Van der Kerkhof, P. C. M. (1986). *Textbook of Psoriasis*. (Edinburgh: Churchill Livingstone)

Index